HUMAN ANATOMY AND PHYSIOLOGY

Additional books in this series can be found on Nova's website under the Series tab.

Additional e-books in this series can be found on Nova's website under the e-book tab.

HUMAN ANATOMY AND PHYSIOLOGY

FISTULAS AND FISSURES

TYPES, SYMPTOMS, CAUSES, AND TREATMENT

HUMAN ANATOMY AND PHYSIOLOGY

FISTULAS AND FISSURES

TYPES, SYMPTOMS, CAUSES, AND TREATMENT

DMITRI PAVLOVICH
AND
SERGEI IVANOVICH
EDITORS

New York

For permission to use material from this book please contact us:
Telephone 631-231-7269; Fax 631-231-8175
Web Site: http://www.novapublishers.com

NOTICE TO THE READER

Additional color graphics may be available in the e-book version of this book.

Library of Congress Cataloging-in-Publication Data

ISBN: 978-1-62618-068-0

Library of Congress Control Number: 2013931035

Published by Nova Science Publishers, Inc. † New York

Contents

PREFACE

In this book, the authors present current research in the study of the types, symptoms and treatments for fistulas and fissures. Topics include pancreatic fistulas; cutaneous advancement flap combined with tailored lateral internal sphincterotomy for chronic anal fissures; management of congenital fistulae; foot fissures in patients with diabetes; dialysis access-associated steal syndrome; anal fissures; advantage of surgical treatment for intracranial dural arteriovenous fistulas; pathogenesis of perianal fistulas in Crohn's disease; setons in treatment of anal fistulas; biliary fistulas; and arm fistulae and their creation.

Chapter 1 - Pancreatic fistula is a common complication after pancreatic resections, its incidence ranges from 10 to 30 % in most series. It is not a life-threatening complication in most cases; however, it prolongs the hospital stay, increases the treatment costs and delays adjuvant therapy in malignant disease.

Various definitions of pancreatic fistula have been proposed, they are mostly based on the volume, duration, and amylase concentrations of fluid in perioperatively or postoperatively placed drains. It makes comparison of the results difficult. Thus it is advisable to use a uniform definition of the pancreatic fistula and the definition of the ISGPF seems to be optimal. This universal definition is nowadays widely accepted and used. ISGPF defines pancreatic fistula as output via an operatively placed drain (or a subsequently placed percutaneous drain) of any measurable volume of drain fluid on or after postoperative day 3, with an amylase content greater than 3 times the upper normal serum value. The fistula is then graded according to the clinical impact in grades A, B, and C.

There are known three main risk factor categories for the development of pancreatic fistula: related to the pancreatic disease, related to the patient, and related to the surgical procedure. Most of the risk factors for the development of pancreatic fistula cannot be influenced. There are two basic options for the prevention of pancreatic fistula: pharmacological intervention (administration of somatostatin and its analogues) and technical modifications of the pancreatic remnant treatment. Routine administration of octreotide is not advisable in all pancreatic surgical procedures. Rather selective administration in high risk cases is suitable. The second option is modification of pancreatic remnant treatment. Most of the studies studying various modifications of the pancreatic remnant treatment were retrospective with lower level of evidence. There were only a few properly designed randomized trials and they did not prove benefit of one method over another. Besides the technique, the results depend on the experience of surgical department and above all experience of an individual surgeon who performs the pancreatic resection.

The therapy of pancreatic fistula is based on the clinical severity. Fistulas grades A and B according to the ISGPF are always treated conservatively. The patients with fistula grade C usually require intensive care, they are in sepsis, and have failure of one or more organs. The clinical condition requires miniinvasive drainage of the peripancreatic collections or re-operation. There are two basic strategies for the reoperations: surgical drainage of the collections or completing total pancreatectomy. Total pancreatectomy was preferred in the past, however this procedure is technically very demanding with high mortality. Nowadays most of the authors prefer surgical drainage; this procedure is technically less demanding, has lower mortality, the endocrine function of pancreas is protected, and the patients usually need no further interventions.

In conclusion, postoperative pancreatic fistula remains to be a significant problem in pancreatic surgery. The research nowadays continues with the goal to lower the incidence of pancreatic fistula; new techniques and interventions are tested in number of clinical trials.

Chapter 2 - Lateral internal sphincterotomy (LIS) is considered the surgical treatment of choice for chronic idiopathic anal fissure. Except for minor episodes of impaired continence, LIS routinely does not include wound closure, which may lead to complications of secondary wound healing (anal stenosis, keyhole deformity). Flap techniques have the advantage of the primary wound healing avoiding scar formation as a risk for minor anal incontinence. Primary wound healing after fissurectomy is usually impossible owing to increased tension on the suture lines and can only be achieved by a tension-free skin graft. Although no difference has been proven between the two techniques, a lack of data exists on the results of a combined procedure.

Over a period of 3 years, 45 patients who underwent LIS + dermal flap were recruited and prospectively followed-up for a minimum of 6 months. Following a "tailored" LIS (internal sphincter division "up to the level of the fissure apex" a fissurectomy was undertaken. The hypertrophic papilla when present was excised, and the sides of the fissure were freshened by sharp scalpel dissection. A modified, trapezoid-like Y-V flap, consisted of skin and subcutaneous fat, was dissected free of the fibers of the subcutaneous external anal sphincter to allow tension-free advancement into the fissure base. The advanced flap was sutured to the site of the previous fissure.

All except one patient healed completely within 30 days from operation. The intensity of pain post-defecation was reduced significantly compared to the preoperative values even from the first defecation ($p<0.0001$). None of the patients complained of pain at the end of the first postoperative week. Analgesics were not required beyond the 3rd POD. Episodes of minor bleeding occurred in 8 patients in during the period of the first 2 weeks. The only remarkable complication recorded postoperatively was a partial break down occurred in one case, which was managed conservatively. At the 6 months follow-up appointment, no recurrences were recorded and in no case was further surgery necessary. After a median follow-up of 20 months (range 8-36), when all patients were contacted by phone, no patient reported pain or clinical symptoms of anal fissure.

Review of the literature and current results support that flap techniques have the advantage of primary wound healing avoiding scar formation as a risk for minor anal incontinence. The addition of a dermal flap after LIS results in excellent healing and minimal postoperative discomfort. Even though it extends the operative time, at the authors academic clinical practice, the authors have completely changed their therapeutic strategy, incorporating the flap in all cases of surgically treated fissures.

Chapter 3 - Congenital fistulae are separate and distinct from other fistulae as they result from aberrant embryological development rather than from inflammatory processes. Recent developments particularly in minimally invasive surgery have resulted in a paradigm shift in the management and outcome of the varied expression of this condition.

Abnormal connections between the trachea and oesophagus represent one of the archetypical conditions of paediatric surgery. Management of *Tracheo-oesophageal fistula* has improved from a lethal anomaly 60 years ago to the vast majority surviving today. H type fistulas represent an interesting subclass, where there is no associated oesophageal atresia, these can present later with recurrent aspirations and respiratory insults. Thoracoscopy is increasingly being used to manage these fistulae and the authors present current trends in the management of these cases.

Branchial fistulae have a more subtle presentation with a small opening evident most commonly in the anterior triangle of the neck. The precise site of the opening is related to the underlying embryological arch which is involved in the fistulas development. The authors will describe the embryology of these lesions and some recent innovations in surgical approaches to their excision.

The *vitello intestinal duct* usually closes during development, but remnants are often encountered in surgical practice. These maybe present as internal or external structures or as a patent fistula between the ileum and umbilicus. Occasionally, persistence of the vitellointestinal duct may present as an emergency with acute intestinal obstruction from volvulus or an intussusception. Laparoscopy has proven to be a useful adjunct in the elective and acute management of this condition.

Similarly, a *patent urachus* which usually manifests at birth with urine leakage from the umbilicus is amenable to a minimally invasive approach.

Chapter 4 - Fissures in the foot, especially in the heel, are a cause of diabetic foot ulcers, and thus it is important to prevent foot fissures in patients with diabetes. It is known that autonomic neuropathy results in reduced sweat secretion leading to fissures and ulcers. Deep fissures that extend into the dermis may have a particularly higher risk of ulceration than superficial fissures because of damaged skin barrier function. However, factors related to deep fissures are unknown. Therefore, factors related to deep fissures of patients with diabetes were investigated, and the following results were obtained. The prevalence of deep foot fissures was 3.8% in patients with diabetes, with 85.7% of the fissures located in the heel. Autonomic neuropathy and angiopathy were related to deep fissures. It is noteworthy that angiopathy was a newly identified factor related to deep fissures. Next, whether angiopathy causes sweat gland atrophy of the heel skin in diabetic patients was examined. It was found that the number of sweat pores in the heel skin was significantly lower in diabetic patients with angiopathy on microscopic examination of the skin, suggesting that sweat gland atrophy may occur in the heel skin in this population. These results may indicate a loss of tissue durability at the same depth as the sweat glands. Therefore, not only use of moisturizers, but enhancement of the blood supply and external force control might be effective for preventing foot fissures in patients with diabetes.

Chapter 5 - A pancreatic fistula (PF) is an abnormal communication between the pancreatic duct and neighboring organs or spaces. They are classified as external or internal depending on whether they communicate with the skin or other organs.

PFs are caused mainly by acute or chronic pancreatitis, as well as by pancreatic surgery. Their clinical manifestations vary according to their location, size and affected organs, and they may include electrolyte imbalance, malnutrition, infection, abdominal pain, ascites, dyspnea and thoracic pain.

PFs are suspected by clinical features and radiological imaging, and confirmed by the finding of high levels of amylase in the extravasated fluid, which often exceed 4000 U/L. Magnetic resonance cholangiopancreatography should be the first imaging tool used in the diagnostic work-up, followed by endoscopic retrograde cholangiopancreatography, which is the most accurate method but has the drawback of its invasive nature.

The initial treatment of pancreatic fistulae is conservative, including nasojejunal feeding, broad spectrum antibiotic therapy and correction of electrolyte imbalances. This approach achieves closure rates of up to 80 percent.

When conservative therapy fails, endoscopic ERCP treatment is to be employed with the intention to drain collections if present, dilate pancreatic duct strictures and/or reduce pancreatic duct pressure through stent placement.

Surgery is the final option when other approaches prove themselves unsuccessful. Surgical techniques include pancreatic resection and jejunostomy, and achieve success rates of up to 90 percent, with mortality rates of 6 percent in some series.

Chapter 6 - The steal phenomenon is a rarely seen multifactorial complication after hemodialysis access creation. The clinical pictures of steal are variants from mild pain or coldness of distal hand (stage I) to severe tissue necrosis or gangrene (stage IV). The reported incidence ranges from 1.6% to 11%. The occurrences are higher in patients with distal prosthetic graft, side-to-side anastomosis of AV fistula, Diabeties Mellitus, hypertension, coronary artery disease, and female gender. The diagnosis is largely based on the clinical presentations but a varety of methods have been used to confirm the ischemic steal, which include color duplex ultrasound, digital photoplethysmography, pulse oxymetry, and even the infrared thermography. When the steal is suspected, an urgent vascular evaluation and prompt revision of treatment are of the essence. The pathophysiologies of steal syndrome are also various including too large shunting, increased vascular resistance peripheral to the fistula, inflow stenosis, and distal arteriopathy. The goal of treatment is to restore the distal perfusion and to maintain the access function. Many procedures are reported in the literature including access ligation, banding, correction of the inflow lesion, proximalization of arterial inflow (PAI), revision using distal inflow (RUDI), distal revascularization with interval ligation (DRIL), banding between dialysis puncture sites, minimally invasive limited ligation endoluminal-assisted revision (MILLER) banding procedure, ulnar artery dilation, transcatheter collateral veins coil embolization, and ligation of the perforating vein. Because different pathophysiologies present in different patients, the authors discuss and compare the many interventional strategies based on conditions of the proximal arterial stenosis, distal arterial stenosis, low-flow steal syndrome, high-flow steal syndrome, and individual specific situation.

Chapter 7 - Anal fissures are common proctologic problems, associated with significant morbidity. Careful clinical evaluation to distinguish primary from secondary anal fissure is mandatory.

Anal fissure may have underlying pathology such as Crohn's disease, the prevalence of this disease significantly increased in the western countries in the last decades. Cancer and syphilis are other possible underlying diseases.

It is also important to distinguish anal fissures with high anal tone from those with normal anal tone.

Low anal tone and secondary soiling can provoke anoderm laceration which can mimic anal fissure, in this case chemical or surgical sphincterotomy may aggravate the anoderm injury.

Surgical and chemical sphincterotomy are both accepted treatments for chronic anal fissure. No single treatment is best choice for all patients. Both treatments modalities are much improved in the last decades. The authors use now combination and sequential pharmacotherapy e.g. calcium blockers, nitric oxide donors and botulinum toxin on one hand. On the other hand new surgical approaches providing lower risk of incontinence compared to the past and high healing rate. Impairment of anal sphincter by surgical procedure may cause immediate and delayed incontinence. On the other hand pharmacotherapy is much slower treatment modality with higher recurrence rate and increased risk for fissure infection and fistula formation.

Therefore treatment for anal fissure has to be tailored to the individual patients, taking in consideration the level of pain, and the potential individual risk for incontinence.

Chapter 8 - *Overview:* Dural arteriovenous fistulas (AVF) are relative infrequent neurovascular diseases. Since they have abnormal pathways between dural arteries and draining veins, venous infarction or intracerebral hemorrhage (ICH) can be caused by venous congestion. Pathophysiology and etiology are different between arteriovenous malformation (AVM) and AVF. Besides, pathogenesis of dural AVF yet remains unclear. They are usually treated with endovascular surgery. However, transarterial or transvenous embolization often fails to obliterate AVF completely due to cumbersome access and angiographically occult fistulas, which may result in recurrence. Therefore, direct surgery is also important modality for achieving complete therapeutic cure. Here the authors describe the advantages of direct surgery and review previous literatures including their clinical experience.

Role of Direct surgery for Intracranial AVF: Spinal AVFs can be favorably ligated with direct surgery. If intracranial, most of AVFs in the anterior cranial fossa are treated with craniotomy due to difficulty and risk of endovascular approach. On the other hands, direct surgeries for other locations are rarely reported, especially if main drainers were Sylvian vein or deep venous systems such as basal vein of Rosenthal. In these contexts, some cases underwent craniotomy following endovascular surgeries ended in fail. If the fistulas were successfully obliterated, the symptoms improved dramatically. Advantage of open surgery is considered that fistular points and microvessels on the dura can be cauterized and obliterated directly. Further surgical experience is demanded for adequate evidence to expand the validity of direct surgery for the intracranial AVFs.

Pial Fistula: Pial fistulas are rare vascular malformations. The structure of pial fistula is single channel between artery and venous system on the cortex without interventing abnormal vessels (e.g. nidus). As they can cause recurrence unless adequately occluded, potential existence of the pial fistula should be taken care. Conventional digital subtraction angiography (DSA) can hardly identify the pial fistulas, nevertheless, it is usually impossible to obliterate them via endovascular route. Therefore direct surgery plays a quite important role for detection and obliteration of pial fistulas.

Intraoperative Indocyanine Green (ICG) videoangiography for AVF: Currently intraoperative ICG videoangiography has become an indispensable tool for surgeries of several neurovascular lesions. It provides high resolution images of blood flow intraoperatively. For dural AVFs, ICG videoangiography can visualize not only the microvasculature but also residual pial fistulas.

Conclusion and Prospect: Complete detection and obliteration of fistular points, as well as, preservation of normal blood flow are recommended for the treatment of intracranial dural AVFs. The authors believe craniotomy is one of the most favorable treatments for these purposes. Additionally it enables us to obtain specimens of the dura containing fistula and microvasculature, which can develop the understanding about the pathophysiology of AVF. Finally the progress of intraoperative monitoring including ICG videoangiography will provide safe and accurate surgery and has a potential to study flow dynamics of dural AVF for appropriate therapeutic strategy. New generation of ICG videoangiography (FLOW800, Carl Zeiss) will be able to analyze flow dynamics of these vascular malformations.

Chapter 9 - Crohn's disease is a chronic inflammatory disorder that can affect any part of the gastrointestinal tract from the mouth to the anus. The disease is characterized by transmural inflammation that can be complicated by the development of fibrotic strictures, perforation, abscess formation, and fistulization. Perianal fistula is a significant clinical sign in cases with Crohn's disease, which may arise from inflamed or infected anal glands (fistula-in-ano) and/or penetration of fissures or ulcers of the rectum or anal canal. Transmural extension and gut flora play crucial role in the progress and development of Crohn's anal fistulas. The retrieved Escherichia Coli strains from Crohn's disease patients are able to adhere to and to invade intestinal epithelium. They are then capable to survive digestion by the submucosal neutrophils and macrophages.

Persistent infection in Crohn's anal fistulas is mainly due to overproduction of IL-1, IL-6 and TNFα, which are produced by activated macrophages, to poor response to IL-4 and to lack of production of IL-10. This overproduction is further enhanced by the availability of free zinc and the then overproduction of interferon gamma. This likely explains the failure of the concomitant antibiotics Ciprofloxacin for 12 weeks in 24 patients to improve the response to infliximab.

Cyclosporine, Tacrolimus, Azathioprine and 6- Mercaptopurine were all used in treating Crohn's anal fistulas but the outcome was not so successful as it was with infliximab. This is likely because that these thiopurines are mainly acting against activated T Lymphocytes and its productions which play less important role than those produced by activated macrophages.

Although IL-10 is zinc-dependent the provision of zinc would add no benefit. Recombinant IL-10 may offer better chances for better rates of success.

Chapter 10 - High trans-sphincteric fistulas, involving the upper two-thirds of the external sphincter, remain a surgical challenge because incontinence may result from the division of muscle involving more than one-third of the sphincter. The principles of anal fistula surgery are to eliminate the fistula, prevent recurrence and preserve sphincter function.

In contrast with fistulotomy for low anal fistulas, a well-accepted, simple, safe, and efficient method is still lacking for high anal fistulas. Seton techniques still occupy an important position in the treatment of high anal fistulas. The seton works by several mechanisms: (1) it helps in draining pus and controlling sepsis prior to definitive treatment; (2) it stimulates fibrosis and acts as a marker of the fistula tract for sphincter sparing procedures such as fistula plug, fibrin glue and ligation of intersphincteric fistula tract (LIFT); and (3) the tight (cutting) seton promotes slow transection of the external sphincter muscle as a result of pressure necrosis with minimal separation of the cut ends.

Long-term seton drainage is a simple and efficient procedure in treating high anal fistulas in Crohn's disease. This article describes the current options available for management of anal fistula with setons. When a patient presents with anal fistula, it is important to determine the level of fistula, involvement of sphincters (high vs low transphincteric), abscess or local sepsis and the etiology. For low fistula involving less than a third of the sphincters, primary fistulotomy can be performed. For high transphincteric fistula with abscess and local sepsis, a loose seton to act as drainage seton or a drainage tube seton should be placed. Once the abscess has resolved than for a crypt glandular fistula the treatment decision involves the use of sphincter sparing vs sphincter cutting options. Setons for such treatment can be considered either as a cutting or loose seton after discussing the individual merits with the patients. Cutting seton can be used as a single stage or multi-stage procedure. Currently cutting setons are not in much use in the developed countries because of the pain associated with treatment, uncontrolled cutting of sphincter muscles and a higher rate of incontinence. If the patient is willing to try for a prolonged treatment option then he can be offered the long term loose seton. For patients who want to opt for sphincter saving surgery the loose setons are generally left in the fistula tract for 4-6 weeks. Also patient who had started on long term loose seton, but did not want to continue with loose seton, can be considered for one of the sphincter sparing surgery.

Patients with Crohn's disease have a higher risk of recurrence. Once the perianal sepsis is controlled with loose drainage setons/ drainage tubes, consideration should be given for treatment with biological agents such as infliximab. After the disease and sepsis is under control these patient can choose between long term loose seton or sphincter sparing surgeries.

Chapter 11 - Biliary fistulas are uncommon but important causes of significant morbidity and mortality, especially in the elderly patient. The classification of biliary fistulas and the clinical scenarios presented by patients with biliary fistulas have changed over the last two decades following the widespread application of operations on the biliary tract, from laparoscopic cholecystectomy to advanced hepato-biliary surgery to liver transplantation. In addition, there has been a dramatic expansion of non-surgical treatment modalities for biliary disease from both the endoscopic and interventional radiology approach. As a result, these new treatment modalities have not only remarkably improved the treatment of biliary disease, but also introduced new complications, including biliary fistulas, which have been recently described. Early recognition and prompt management of biliary fistulas are essential steps for an effective treatment and to reduce mortality. In addition, the treatment of chronic underlying infection and the maintenance of an adequate nutritional support are critical steps in the management of these often debilitated patients. In this review the authors present an updated classification of biliary fistulas based on current pathophysiology and describe the different clinical scenarios presented by patients with biliary fistulas. The authors also emphasize key aspects in the multidisciplinary approach to these patients and highlight current diagnostic and treatment strategies.

Chapter 12 - The autogenous arterio-venous fistula (AVF) is the gold standard in establishing long-term vascular access in end stage renal disease (ESRD) and can be established in the majority of patients as a day case under local anaesthetic. General anaesthesia is typically only required for more complicated, secondary procedures. Pre-operative clinical examination and duplex ultrasonography are essential in planning vascular access procedures and thus maximising the chances of the fistula being useful for long-term dialysis.

It is imperative that "Venous real estate" be utilised in a careful manner. Peripheral veins should be preserved in all patients (especially those at risk of requiring future renal replacement therapy) by avoiding unnecessary venesection or cannulation. Fistulae should be constructed as distally as possible thus maximising the number of sites that can be used. The most distal fistula should be performed preferably in the non-dominant upper limb.

If possible centrally placed double-lumen catheters and prosthetic grafts should be avoided because of their relatively high complication rates. However, both have roles to play in the management of renal failure patients especially in the emergent situation or when autogenous methods are no longer possible.

The snuff-box fistula is an ideal first fistula. It can be constructed in half of all patients and has good patency rates. The construction of this fistula, the brachio-cephalic and transposed brachial vein fistulae are discussed in this chapter.

In: Fistuals and Fissures
Editors: Dmitri Pavlovich and Sergei Ivanovich

ISBN: 978-1-62618-068-0

Chapter 1

PANCREATIC FISTULA

Filip Čečka* and Bohumil Jon
Department of Surgery,
Medical Faculty and University Hospital Hradec Králové,
Czech Republic

ABSTRACT

Pancreatic fistula is a common complication after pancreatic resections, its incidence ranges from 10 to 30 % in most series. It is not a life-threatening complication in most cases; however, it prolongs the hospital stay, increases the treatment costs and delays adjuvant therapy in malignant disease.

Various definitions of pancreatic fistula have been proposed, they are mostly based on the volume, duration, and amylase concentrations of fluid in perioperatively or postoperatively placed drains. It makes comparison of the results difficult. Thus it is advisable to use a uniform definition of the pancreatic fistula and the definition of the ISGPF seems to be optimal. This universal definition is nowadays widely accepted and used. ISGPF defines pancreatic fistula as output via an operatively placed drain (or a subsequently placed percutaneous drain) of any measurable volume of drain fluid on or after postoperative day 3, with an amylase content greater than 3 times the upper normal serum value. The fistula is then graded according to the clinical impact in grades A, B, and C.

There are known three main risk factor categories for the development of pancreatic fistula: related to the pancreatic disease, related to the patient, and related to the surgical procedure. Most of the risk factors for the development of pancreatic fistula cannot be influenced. There are two basic options for the prevention of pancreatic fistula: pharmacological intervention (administration of somatostatin and its analogues) and technical modifications of the pancreatic remnant treatment. Routine administration of octreotide is not advisable in all pancreatic surgical procedures. Rather selective administration in high risk cases is suitable. The second option is modification of pancreatic remnant treatment. Most of the studies studying various modifications of the

* Corresponding Author: Filip Čečka MD PhD, Department of Surgery, Faculty of Medicine and University Hospital Hradec Králové, Sokolská 581, 500 05 Hradec Králové, Czech Republic, tel.: ++420-737-163931, fax: ++420-495-832026, e-mail: filip.cecka@seznam.cz.

pancreatic remnant treatment were retrospective with lower level of evidence. There were only a few properly designed randomized trials and they did not prove benefit of one method over another. Besides the technique, the results depend on the experience of surgical department and above all experience of an individual surgeon who performs the pancreatic resection.

The therapy of pancreatic fistula is based on the clinical severity. Fistulas grades A and B according to the ISGPF are always treated conservatively. The patients with fistula grade C usually require intensive care, they are in sepsis, and have failure of one or more organs. The clinical condition requires miniinvasive drainage of the peripancreatic collections or re-operation. There are two basic strategies for the reoperations: surgical drainage of the collections or completing total pancreatectomy. Total pancreatectomy was preferred in the past, however this procedure is technically very demanding with high mortality. Nowadays most of the authors prefer surgical drainage; this procedure is technically less demanding, has lower mortality, the endocrine function of pancreas is protected, and the patients usually need no further interventions.

In conclusion, postoperative pancreatic fistula remains to be a significant problem in pancreatic surgery. The research nowadays continues with the goal to lower the incidence of pancreatic fistula; new techniques and interventions are tested in number of clinical trials.

1. Introduction

Pancreatic fistula (PF) is a condition which occurs mainly after pancreatic resections, traumatic injury of the pancreas, or injury of the pancreas during surgery of nearby organs. In general, it is caused by the leakage of pancreatic juice into the retroperitoneum or abdominal cavity.

Pancreatic resection is the most common cause of the pancreatic fistula. The mortality associated with this procedure has decreased rapidly in the past decades due to refinements in operative technique, introduction of new surgical devices, and improvements in postoperative care including new interventional radiology techniques [1]. However, the morbidity remains high [2]. The main reason for postoperative morbidity is the postoperative pancreatic fistula, which is also regarded as the most ominous complication following pancreatic resection [3]. PF is not a life-threatening condition in most cases; however it prolongs the hospital stay, increases the cost of the treatment and delays adjuvant treatment in malignant disease [4]. PF remains a significant issue, mainly in modern pancreatic surgery.

2. Causes and Definition of PF

PF is generally defined as an abnormal connection between the pancreatic duct epithelium and another epithelial surface containing pancreas-derived, enzyme-rich fluid [5]. PF is caused by exocrine secretion from the remnant pancreatic parenchyma, therefore output of a liquid rich in amylase content is considered to be a defining feature of PF [3]. Failure of healing the pancreaticoenteric anastomosis or leak from the suture of the pancreatic parenchyma after distal pancreatectomy, central pancreatectomy or enucleation causes the subsequent complications. Pancreatic juice is rich in protease, which after activation causes digestion of peripancreatic tissue, its destruction, and in cases of pancreaticoenteric anastomosis causes dehiscence of the anastomosis. Additional digestion and destruction of the surrounding tissue may be followed by the development of peripancreatic fluid collections, intra-abdominal or retroperitoneal abscesses, delayed gastric emptying, and postoperative hemorrhage.

The reported incidence of PF varies in the surgical literature from 10% to over 30% [6]. This wide variability is largely due to different definitions of pancreatic fistula [7]. Most of the definitions are based on the volume, duration, and amylase concentrations in perioperatively or postoperatively placed drains. When various definitions of pancreatic fistula are applied to identical groups of patients, the rate of pancreatic fistula can range from 10% to 29% according to the definition which is applied [7].

A new universal definition of pancreatic fistula was published in 2005 [5]. According to the International Study Group on Pancreatic Fistula (ISGPF), pancreatic fistula is defined as output via an operatively placed drain (or a subsequently placed percutaneous drain) of any measurable volume of drain fluid on or after postoperative day 3, with an amylase content greater than three times the upper normal serum value [5]. Three grades of pancreatic fistula were determined according to the clinical severity as A, B, or C [Table 1].

Grade A fistula, also called "transient fistula" has no clinical impact. It requires little or no change in the clinical management of the patient. Grade A fistula is not associated with a delay in hospital discharge; however, the patients may be discharged with the drain. The drains are usually removed within 3 weeks. Imaging studies do not reveal worrisome or suspicious peripancreatic collections.

Grade B fistulas are symptomatic and clinically apparent, and they require changes in clinical management or adjustment of the clinical pathway. The patients are usually supported by enteral or parenteral nutrition, and the peripancreatic drains are usually kept in place or new drains may be inserted. The patients may have abdominal pain, fever, and leukocytosis.

Grade C fistulas are severe and clinically significant, and they require major adjustments in clinical management. Clinical intervention is aggressive; patients are often placed in the intensive care units (ICU) and have enteral or parenteral nutrition, antibiotics, and somatostatin analogues. A CT scan usually shows worrisome peripancreatic fluid collection(s) that require percutaneous drainage. Surgical revision may be indicated in some cases.

Table 1. Pancreatic fistula definition according to the ISGPF [5]

Grade	A	B	C
Clinical condition	Well	Often well	Ill appearing/bad
Specific treatment	No	Yes/no	Yes
US/CT	Negative	Negative/positive	Positive
Persistent drainage (after 3 weeks)	No	Usually yes	Yes
Reoperation	No	No	Yes
Death related to PF	No	No	Possibly yes
Signs of infection	No	Yes	Yes
Sepsis	No	No	Yes
Readmission	No	Yes/no	Yes/no

The incidence of pancreatic fistula after pancreaticoduodenectomy and distal pancreatectomy have been equally reported in several studies [8]. Nevertheless, the clinical significance of pancreatic fistula after pancreaticoduodenectomy or distal pancreatectomy is different. Sauvanet suggested that pancreatic fistula originating from pancreaticoenteric anastomosis seems to have worse prognosis than pancreatic fistula originating from a pancreatic remnant [9]. This may be due to the activation of pancreatic juice by enterokinase, which is a necessary mechanism that stimulates the procteoclastic activity of various pancreatic enzymes [10]. This process may contribute to the differences between pancreatic fistulas after operations that require enteric reconstructions (pancreaticoduodenectomy and central pancreatic resection) and those that do not (distal pancreatectomy and enucleation). Pratt suggested that clinically relevant fistulas after pancreaticoduodenectomy require more aggressive management in intensive care settings compared to those that occur after distal resections. Surgical exploration, when indicated, is more often urgent. On the other hand, fistulas that occur after distal resections often require prolonged drainage of intra-abdominal collections and multiple hospital readmissions, usually for image-guided percutaneous drainage [8].

3. Risk Factors of Development of PF

There are many risk factors associated with the development of PF. They can be divided into the following categories: 1/ factors associated with the pancreas, 2/ factors associated with the patient, and 3/ factors associated with the surgical procedure.

3.1. Factors Associated with the Pancreas

The main risk factor for PF is the structure of the pancreatic parenchyma. Soft pancreatic texture has been widely recognized as the most important risk factor for development of PF [11]. A large series of nearly 2000 pancreaticoduodenectomies showed a fistula rate of 22 % in soft pancreas, whereas no patient with a firm gland developed a PF [11]. Other authors reported similar rates of PF in the presence of soft pancreatic parenchyma [6, 12]. The soft and friable pancreatic parenchyma makes the anastomosis difficult to perform. On the other hand, hard fibrotic pancreatic remnant in patients with chronic pancreatitis facilitates the construction of anastomosis.

Another major predictor of PF development is the size of the main pancreatic duct. A small, non-dilated duct is an important risk factor for PF in comparison to a large, dilated duct [3, 13]. Important is also the pathological lesion, for which is the pancreatic resection performed; ampullary and duodenal carcinoma, distal bile duct carcinoma, and endocrine tumors have higher rates of PF [11], because the pancreatic parenchyma is soft with a small main pancreatic duct in these conditions.

3.2. Factors Associated with the Patient

Certain characteristics predispose the patients to a higher risk of PF development; these include an age over 70 years [14], male gender [11], patients with a history of ischemic heart disease [11], patients with increased body-mass index [15]. The ischemic heart disease may cause lower visceral perfusion and thus compromise pancreatic anastomosis healing. Another risk factor is preoperative duration of jaundice rather than the absolute level of bilirubin [16]. PF was associated with a significantly lower creatinine clearance in the same study [16]. This may be explained by the theory that lower creatinine clearance may precipitate acute renal failure, intra-abdominal bleeding, and sepsis. The role of diabetes mellitus is not yet clear. However, most studies showed diabetes to be a risk factor for PF formation [17-19].

3.3. Factors Associated with the Surgical Procedure

Risk factors associated with the surgical procedure include technical modifications of the surgical procedure and the pharmacological interventions (mentioned below). Other minor risk factors include greater blood loss, longer operating time, and resections of adjacent organs. Greater blood loss has been shown to correlate with a greater incidence of PF in several studies [17, 20, 21]. Some authors claim that the increased blood loss is likely to be associated with other risk factors including more advanced stages of the disease [16]. A longer operating time has been shown to correlate with an increased incidence of PF but the correlation did not reach statistical significance [21]. Patients with multivisceral pancreatic resection also are at greater risk of PF than patients with a standard pancreatic resection [21]. It might be speculated that extensive multivisceral resections compromise the healing of the pancreatic remnant. Another possible explanation could be a reduced blood supply at the cut surface of the pancreas due to the extent of the resection [21]. On the other hand, preoperative chemoradiotherapy has been showed to decrease the risk of PF [22]. This may be explained by a decrease in pancreatic exocrine secretion caused by the radiotherapy.

The experience of the pancreatic surgery center and especially of the surgeon who performs the pancreatic resection is of great importance. Schmidt analyzed outcomes of pancreaticoduodenectomy in 1003 patients according to surgeon experience and volume. Surgeons who performed 50 or more pancreaticoduodenectomies were defined as experienced surgeons. Surgeons who performed fewer than 50 pancreaticoduodenectomies were defined as less experienced surgeons. Compared with the less experienced surgeons, experienced surgeons performed pancreaticoduodenectomy with a lower morbidity and lower rate of PF. The mortality was comparable in both groups [23]. Surgeon volume was defined as the number of pancreaticoduodenectomies performed annually by an individual surgeon. Low-volume surgeons were defined as performing fewer than 20 pancreaticoduodenectomies per year; high-volume surgeons were defined as performing 20 or more pancreaticoduodenectomies per year. Low-volume surgeons performed pancreaticoduodenectomy with statistically equivalent mortality, morbidity and pancreatic fistula compared with high-volume surgeons in this study [23]. Similar results were shown comparing the outcomes of pancreaticoduodenectomies in high-volume and low-volume pancreatic surgery centers; the mortality rates in particular are significantly lower in the high-volume centers [24, 25].

4. Preventive Approaches

Pancreatic fistula has significant clinical and economic consequences; it increases the postoperative mortality, prolongs the hospital stay, increases the cost of the treatment, requires the use of other examination and therapeutic interventions, and delays the commencement of adjuvant treatment in malignant disease [4, 26]. It is thus necessary to attempt to lower the PF rate by all available measures. Unfortunately, most of the above-mentioned risk factors cannot be influenced. There are basically only two possible options to lower the rates of PF: pharmacological interventions and technical modifications of the pancreatic remnant management.

4.1. Pharmacological Interventions

The pharmacological approach to prevent anastomotic leak after pancreatic surgery was first described by a German group who reported a reduced morbidity after pancreaticoduodenectomy with perioperative infusion of somatostatin [27]. Preliminary data from this study suggested that continuous infusion of somatostatin reduced the rate of pancreas-specific complications after pancreaticoduodenectomy.

Somatostatin-14, a 14 amino acid hormone, is a potent inhibitor of gastrointestinal secretion. It inhibits both endocrine and exocrine pancreatic secretion. In addition, somatostatin-14 has been shown to have additional effects in reducing gastrointestinal motility, gastric secretion, gall bladder emptying, and pancreatic blood flow [28]. In theory, the physiological characteristics were thought to have a considerable impact on the prevention of pancreas-related complications after pancreatic surgery. The inhibition of gastrointestinal secretion would reduce the volume of secreted fluid as well as the content of the pancreatic enzymes. In addition, the reduced blood flow would possibly diminish the risk of serious hemorrhage. On the other hand, the reduced blood flow could have a negative effect on the healing of the pancreatic anastomosis.

However, the short half-life of somatostatin-14 (several minutes) required continuous administration. The synthetic somatostatin analogue octreotide was developed in order to extend the half-life of the native hormone. Octreotide has a half-life of approximately 90 to 120 minutes, thus allowing fractioned subcutaneous administration. Octreotide has a similar mode of action and similar clinical effects as somatostatin-14. It greatly facilitated the clinical application [29]. The effect of other somatostatin analogues, e.g. vapreotide and lanreotide, on exocrine pancreatic secretion have been studied in terms of the potential for treating pancreatic fistulas or preventing fistulas after pancreatic surgery [30, 31].

Ten randomized prospective trials and 6 meta-analyses comparing the effect of somatostatin and its analogues have been published in the world literature. The results are summarized in Table 2. The results of the reviewed trials are inconsistent and often contradictory. The first four European studies were multi-center [32-35]. They included various types of surgical procedures performed by a large number of surgeons in many hospitals, e.g. the trial by Montorsi included 218 patients from 33 surgical departments studied over two years, meaning on average only three patients per center annually.

Table 2. Design and results of the randomized controlled trials

author	year	patients	types of the operations	dg.	pancreatic fistula		morbidity		benefit
					SA	control	SA	control	
		n			%	%	%	%	
Büchler [32]	1992	246	DPE, DP, DPPHR, E, PJ	M, CP	17,6	38	32	55,4	yes
Pederzoli [35]	1994	252	DPE, DP, DPPHR, CPR, E, PJ	M, CP	9	18,5	15,6	29,2	yes
Friess [33]	1995	247	DPE, DP, DPPHR, PJ	CP	9,8	22,4	16,4	29,6	yes
Montorsi [34]	1995	218	DPE, DP, STP, E	M, CP	9	19,6	21,6	36,4	yes
Lowy [36]	1997	110	DPE	M	28,1	20,8	29,8	24,5	no
Yeo [12]	2000	211	DPE	M	10,6	9,3	40,4	33,6	no
Gouillat [38]	2001	75	DPE	M	10,5	27	21,1	35,1	yes
Shan [39]	2003	54	DPE	M	7,4	7,4	25,9	51,9	yes
Sarr [42]	2003	275	DPE, CPR, DP	M	23,7	22,9	30,4	26,4	no
Suc [37]	2004	230	DPE, DP	M, CP	17,2	18,5	22,1	32,4	yes (selective)

DPE (pancreaticoduodenectomy), CPR (central pancreatic resection), DP (distal pancreatectomy), DPPHR (duodenum-preserving pancreatic head resection), E (enucleation), PJ (pancreaticojejunostomy), STP (subtotal pancreatectomy), M (malignancy), CP (chronic pancreatitis), SA (somatostatin and its analogues), dg. (diagnosis).

Montorsi [34] and Friess [33] showed a significant decrease in the rate of pancreatic fistula, and all four trials showed a decrease in the morbidity rate.

The next two randomized trials were conducted in high-volume centers in the USA and brought completely different results. Lowy et al. [36] published the first single-institution randomized prospective study. However, it carries certain disadvantages. First, it was not placebo-controlled. The patients were randomized to receive either octreotide or no treatment. Second, many patients underwent chemoradiation therapy before the operation. The preoperative chemoradiation was associated with a decreased rate of pancreatic leak in univariate analysis. The study by Yeo and colleagues [12] was reported from a high-volume center. It was criticized for its high withdrawal rate of patients not receiving octreotide for five days (n=40), which was due to the logistical and pharmacy issues according to the authors. Furthermore, the study was terminated before it recruited the scheduled number of patients. In the discussion, the author himself admitted that he had expected a negative result at the very outset of the trial.

The differences between the European and American trials may be partly attributable to the different designs of the trials (multi-center vs. single-center), various procedures included in the trials, different dosage and timing of octreotide administration, and also different definitions of pancreatic fistula. It is a well-known fact that the concentration of pancreatic resections in high-volume centers brings better results, lower morbidity and mortality. The fistula rate in the European trials was from 19% to 38%, whereas in the American trials it was 9% and 21%. The mortality rate reported by Montorsi was 6.9% [34], compared to the mortality reported by Yeo of less than 1% [12]. It has been suggested that the use of octreotide is not beneficial in high-volume centers, where the rate of pancreatic fistula is already rather low. It could however be beneficial in low-volume centers with less experienced surgeons.

The study reported by Suc [37] showed that the benefit of octreotide is somewhere between the conclusions of the four European studies and the two American studies. The authors recommend its use only in high-risk patients with soft pancreas and with the diameter of the main pancreatic duct less than 3 mm. According to the authors, the multi-center design of this study makes the result more plausible for the overall surgical population.

Two trials studied the effect of continuous infusion of somatostatin [38, 39]. They were smaller than the other trials (75 and 54 patients, respectively), which may lower the reliability of the conclusions. However, they both demonstrated the benefits of somatostatin. Shan and colleagues [39] calculated the cost of somatostatin for 7 days ($2380) and of octreotide for 7 days ($357). The prophylactic use of somatostatin in this study saved an average of $8234 in patients with complications. According to Shan [39], the administration of somatostatin could have a better effect than the administration of octreotide. Octreotide is a potent inhibitor of pancreatic exocrine secretion but the initial potent inhibition diminishes considerably after several days of application [40]. This adaptation phenomenon does not occur with somatostatin. Furthermore, after continuous infusion of somatostatin, a therapeutic level could be achieved more rapidly and maintained more reliably. The administration of somatostatin is accomplished by continuous infusion via existing access, as the majority of patients receive intravenous medication. Octreotide is administered by subcutaneous injection, which could be painful and less comfortable for the patients. However, the benefit of somatostatin over octreotide was not shown in another trial [41]. Closset and colleagues conducted a randomized controlled trial comparing somatostatin with octreotide in the prevention of complications after pancreaticoduodenectomy. 50 patients were randomized into two groups, 25 treated with somatostatin, 25 with octreotide. The trial did not show any significant difference in the postoperative complications or rate of pancreatic fistula between the two study groups. Only the comparison of lipase and amylase concentrations in peripancreatic surgically placed drains showed a more rapidly decreasing trend in the somatostatin group, but it was not statistically significant. Regarding the treatment cost, the daily cost of octreotide was 10 times lower than the daily cost of somatostatin treatment [41]. Closset claims that the subcutaneous administration of octreotide is more convenient for the hospital staff [41].

Sarr performed the only trial studying the effect of vapreotide [42]. This trial also has its limitations. First, the extent and duration of the inhibition of pancreatic secretion after the administration of vapreotide has not been fully studied in humans. The authors only presumed that the effect of vapreotide would persist for 8 to 12 hours without having any supporting data, and therefore they administered vapreotide twice per day. Second, the authors could not fully exclude the possibility that there was a selection bias by the investigators since very high-risk patients were not asked to enter the study. The effect of vapreotide would have been in fact the most beneficial in the high-risk group. Third, the trial was stopped based on the results of an interim analysis and thus the planned number of patients to be enrolled in the study was not met.

None of the above-mentioned trials showed any decrease in mortality with the use of somatostatin and its analogues. It could be the result of the fact that the mortality was already low even in the control groups in most of the trials. Furthermore, the trials were not originally designed to discriminate on the basis of mortality.

The comparison of the randomized trials is difficult because the trials differ in terms of study design, diagnosis, operative procedures, drug and drug dosage, time of administration, and above all the definitions of postoperative complications and pancreatic fistula. Instead of conducting a meta-analysis, it is advisable to carefully interpret the results of the individual trials in order to achieve valid conclusions [43].

Based on the current knowledge, the routine administration of somatostatin and its analogues in elective pancreatic surgery cannot be recommended. However, selective administration is advisable in cases which carry a significantly higher risk of developing pancreatic fistula. Somatostatin and its analogues may significantly reduce the pancreatic fistula rate after pancreaticoduodenectomy in low-volume centers, performed by low-volume surgeons, especially when the postoperative fistula rate exceeds 10%. Administering somatostatin and its analogues is recommended in high-risk pancreatic glands, e.g. soft pancreas and when the main pancreatic duct diameter is less than 3 mm. On the contrary, it is not recommended in surgery for chronic pancreatitis. It is known that the fistula rate after distal pancreatectomy or enucleations may be higher than after pancreaticoduodenectomy, and thus the administration of somatostatin and its analogues is recommended in these procedures. There is no data showing that the administration of octreotide prior to surgery brings better results than administration after surgery. However, several authors prefer commencement of administration one hour before the surgery to allow downregulation of digestive secretion at the time of the surgical procedure. There is no data showing significant advantages of somatostatin over its analogues in decreasing the rate of pancreatic fistula. However, the cost of treatment with somatostatin is significantly higher than with octreotide [43]. Somatostatin and its analogues do not decrease mortality in elective pancreatic surgery.

4.2. Technical Modifications of Management of the Pancreatic Remnant

Management of the pancreatic parenchyma remnant and its modifications have been extensively studied in order to lower the rate of PF. There are two basic approaches: management of the pancreatic remnant after pancreaticoduodenectomy and the management of the pancreatic remnant after distal pancreatectomy. In addition to the typical resections, enucleation and central pancreatic resections are possible although less common. Enucleation of pancreatic tumors is performed mainly in small endocrine tumors up to 3 cm in diameter. The pancreatic fistula rate after enucleation is higher than after typical resection, but the PF is usually less severe [44]. The risk of PF after enucleation is increased if the main pancreatic duct is less than 2 mm from the tumor, thus typical resection should be preferred in those cases [45]. Central resection of the pancreas is another option, especially for small benign tumors (mostly cystic tumors) in the body of the pancreas [46]. There are two cut-surfaces in the pancreas which double the risk of pancreatic fistula. Management of the proximal remnant is the same is the management of the pancreatic remnant after distal pancreatectomy; and the management of the distal remnant is analogous to the management of the remnant after pancreaticoduodenectomy, e.g. pancreaticojejuno- or pancreaticogastrostomy must be performed. Both procedures are discussed below. The pancreatic fistula rate after central resection can reach 100% even in high-volume centers [8].

4.2.1. Management of the Pancreatic Remnant after Pancreaticoduodenectomy

There are around 80 possible methods of reconstruction after pancreaticoduodenectomy [47]. The following options of the pancreatic remnant management are among the most frequently discussed.

Pancreaticojejunostomy and pancreaticogastrostomy are the two commonly preferred options for pancreatic remnant implantation. Pancreaticojejunostomy is more favored among surgeons and it is performed in 80 % of the cases. A meta-analysis and systematic review published in 2007 included 3 randomized trials and 13 nonrandomized observational studies [48]. Meta-analysis of 3 randomized controlled trials (RCT) revealed no significant difference between pancreaticojejunostomy and pancreaticogastrostomy regarding overall postoperative complications, pancreatic fistula, intra-abdominal fluid collection, or mortality. On the contrary, analysis of 13 nonrandomized observational clinical studies showed significant results in favor of pancreaticogastrostomy for the outcome parameters with a reduction of pancreatic fistula and mortality in favor of pancreaticogastrostomy. The superiority of pancreaticogastrostomy over pancreaticojejunostomy was most likely influenced by publication bias.

A large number of studies have described modifications of the pancreaticojejunostomy, for example anastomosis end-to-end, end-to-side, anastomosis on the separated Roux-en-Y jejunal loop, pancreatic remnant anatomy modifications, etc [3]. The most common modifications are duct-to-mucosa pancreaticojejunostomy and end-to-side one layer pancreaticojejunostomy. Several retrospective observational studies showed that the duct-to-mucosa pancreaticojejunostomy brings better results with lower PF fistula. However, the only RCT did not show benefit of the duct-to-mucosa pancreaticojejunostomy over the end-to-side one layer anastomosis [49]. Other RCTs compared duct-to-mucosa anastomosis with invaginating pancreaticojejunostomy. Berger randomized 197 patients to receive duct-to-mucosa anastomosis and invagination PJ anastomosis and found a lower PF rate in the invagination group [50]. Chou reported a lower rate of PF in the duct-to-mucosa group (4% vs. 15%), although the difference was not statistically significant [51]. Occlusion of the pancreatic duct instead of anastomosis is not considered an option any more [52].

Placement of plastic stents into the pancreaticojejunostomy has been recommended in order to decrease the PF rate. Authors in favor of the stent argue that it facilitates precise placement of mucous sutures, decreases the risk of iatrogenic pancreatic occlusion, and diverts pancreatic juice away from the anastomosis [53]. However, the stent may become obstructed and lead to PF or it may migrate and cause injury to the anastomosis or bowel [54], or acute pancreatitis may be caused when removing the external stents. Internal stents are designed to fall spontaneously into the bowel [54]. External stents are removed in the postoperative course after the risk of pancreatic fistula passes [53]. External stents have the theoretical advantage of more complete diversion of the pancreatic juice. Five randomized studies and a number of observational retrospective studies have been published with conflicting results. Pessauex and Poon showed benefits of external stents. Winter found no benefit of internal stents compared to no stents. Two studies compared internal vs. external stents. Both groups in both studies had comparable outcomes regarding morbidity, PF rate and mortality; however authors in both studies were in favor of internal stents [53, 54]. Authors of a systemic review and meta-analysis conclude that the number of RCT is too small to allow firm conclusions; however, external stents seemed to reduce the PF rate compared to the control.

Other surgical technical modifications which are worth mentioning include the use of magnification. The authors showed on retrospective analysis that the use of surgical microscope decreases the rate of PF [55].

4.2.2. Management of the Pancreatic Remnant after Distal Pancreatectomy

Distal pancreatectomy is a procedure less frequently performed than pancreaticoduodenectomy. It is due to the fact that lesions in the body and tail of the pancreas are less common. Moreover, malignant tumors in the body and tail are more often advanced or disseminated and therefore non-resectable. The most commonly used techniques are manual suture of the pancreatic remnant and the staple closure [21, 56]. Two retrospective cohort studies showed lower rate of PF in the manual suture group [21, 57], while two other studies did not show any difference between either method [56, 58]. A recently published randomized study compared these two methods in a large multi-center study. 450 patients were randomized, 221 patients were treated with a stapler, 229 received a hand-sewn closure. The authors concluded that that the stapler closure did not reduce the PF rate compared to the hand-sewn closure [59].

Besides these two commonly used techniques, others were described, mostly in retrospective cohort analysis. Wagner used Roux-en-Y drainage for the management of the pancreatic remnant. The authors manage to decrease the PF rate; however, the main disadvantage of this technique is greater severity of the fistula when it occurs. Other techniques include patch of the pancreatic remnant with the first jejunal loop, occlusion of the pancreatic remnant with prolamine, a special sandwich method with fibrin glue application before manual suture, etc. [59].

Laparoscopic distal pancreatectomy is considered to be a technically feasible and safe method of treatment of lesions in the body and tail of the pancreas. The benefit of a laparoscopic approach in distal pancreatectomy has been shown in several retrospective studies which were summarized in a review and meta-analysis [60, 61]. The laparoscopic approach has all the advantages of mini-invasive treatment: lower blood loss, shorter hospital stay, lower analgesia consumption in the postoperative period, faster return to normal diet and normal daily activities, better cosmetic results. The disadvantages include a longer operating time, higher cost for the surgical procedure and a long learning curve. Regarding pancreatic fistula, no individual study showed a lower rate of PF in the laparoscopic approach. A systematic review again showed no differences between the open and laparoscopic approach [60]. However, the meta-analysis showed a lower PF rate in the laparoscopic approach [61]. As in the open distal pancreatectomy, the method of pancreatic remnant management is an important factor in the PF rate. But unlike in the open approach, no study has yet compared various methods of management of the pancreatic remnant in laparoscopic distal pancreatectomy. The most commonly used method is the transection of pancreatic parenchyma with a stapler. Various types of staplers are used by various authors; the choice of the stapler is usually based on individual experience rather than evidence. The stapler type should be chosen according to the firmness of the pancreatic parenchyma [62]. For soft pancreas, smaller staples 2.5-3.5mm should be used. For hard fibrotic pancreatic parenchyma, larger staples 3.7-.4.5 mm should be used [62]. One study showed the benefit of vascular staples over other types of staples [63]. Other techniques are used less frequently, e.g. transection of the pancreas with Ligasure, bipolar coagulation, harmonic scalpel, etc. Several authors described better outcomes with fibrin glue applied on the pancreatic remnant. So far there is no consensus on the optimal technique of pancreatic remnant management so far. Individual authors use various techniques based on their discretion rather than evidence. It is difficult to compare results among the studies as various PF definitions are used. However, from the current knowledge, we can conclude that combined techniques of pancreatic remnant management bring better results, e.g. titan clips and fibrin glue applied on the stapler line, or a combination of stapler, manual suture, fibrin glue and omentoplasty [62].

The most effective way to prevent PF after pancreaticoduodenectomy or distal pancreatectomy remains controversial. Most of the conducted randomized studies bring controversial or contradictory results. Current literature shows that while the method of surgical technique is very important, the skill of the operating surgeon, individual experience, and the volume of the center may play an even a greater role [23].

5. Diagnosis of the PF

As pancreatic fistula may become a severe complication after pancreatic resection, all measures must be taken to recognize this condition in the early stages in order to start appropriate therapy as soon as the complication develops. This can help minimize the potentially devastating effects. Most PF occur 3 to 7 days postoperatively [6].

Any deviation in the normal postoperative course of a patient after major pancreatic surgery gives rise to suspicion of the PF development. Clinical signs are usually nonspecific and usually include upper abdominal discomfort, nausea, vomiting, loss of appetite, tender and rigid abdomen, failure to pass stool, dyspnea, tachycardia or other signs of sepsis. Laboratory tests show leukocytosis and increased CRP; serum amylase is not usually elevated. A radiological examination is not necessary in routine setting, although it may be performed in suspicious cases. If done in such cases, it reveals fluid collections in the abdominal cavity, pleural effusion, abscesses in the subphrenic areas or retroperitoneum, or a distended bowel [3]. A CT scan often shows unspecific changes such as pancreatic edema or peripancreatic fluid collections. However, late complications such as abscess formation, or visceral artery pseudoaneurysms are clearly visible [3]. A CT scan is then also a therapeutic modality, as new drains into the peripancreatic fluid collections or intra-abdominal abscesses can be inserted under CT guidance.

The most important diagnostic tool is the evaluation of the effluent from intra-abdominal drains. There can be high fluid output, it can have sinister appearance or the content may be infected [5]. Other complications through which the pancreatic fistula may present include severe wound infection, delayed hemorrhage, or delayed gastric emptying. The index of suspicion is usually higher in patients with several risk factors for development of PF. Amylase concentration of the drain effluent greater than three times the upper limit of normal serum value confirms the diagnosis of PF [5].

Although amylase concentration in the drain output is important in the diagnosis of PF, it is of no use when predicting the severity of PF [64]. Distinguishing clinically significant fistulas (grades B and C) from transient fistulas is an essential question in the early period of the fistula's appearance. The ISGPF classification was developed to retrospectively evaluate the fistula grade. It thus has no value in predicting the severity of the fistula at its outset and it is of no help in clinical decision making. A recent study has focused on factors which would predict the necessity for reoperation and factors linked with higher mortality rates. The authors demonstrated that elevated serum bilirubin and amylase were associated with more severe fistula rates. Furthermore, elevated serum amylase was identified as an independent prognostic factor requiring reoperation, with high C-reactive protein (over 100 mg/l) being identified as an independent prognostic factor associated with increased rates of reoperation [64].

6. THERAPY OF THE PF

The treatment of PF must be individualized according to the clinical condition of the patient; it consists of conservative measures in majority of patients.

PF grade A is clinically non-significant; it has no clinical consequences, does not prolong the hospital stay, nor does it increase the cost of the treatment. The peroperatively placed drains must be kept in place until the amylase-rich fluid secretion resolves, which is usually within 3 weeks after the surgery. No other measures besides keeping the drains in place are necessary [65].

PF grade B requires change in the management, although the treatment remains conservative. It includes enteral or parenteral nutrition as well as antibiotics. Therapeutic somatostatin or its analogues can be also administered to reduce the pancreatic secretion. Peroperatively placed drains must be kept in place. Proper fixation of the drains is crucial in order to prevent their accidental loss. Follow-up CT scans might be useful to reveal new fluid collections or abscess formations. New drains might be inserted to drain any undrained peripancreatic collections. Percutaneous CT-guided drainage significantly reduced the need for relaparotomy [65].

PF grade C is clinically the most severe. The patients usually must be placed in the intensive care unit; they can suffer from sepsis, failure of one or more organs. In case peripancreatic fluid collections are found on CT scan, those are drained under CT-guidance. Only a small group of patients develop abdominal sepsis requiring another surgical procedure. The operative management depends on the clinical condition of the patient, the vitality pancreatic remnant, and the degree of anastomotic dehiscence. Surgical repair of the anastomosis is not attempted in most cases because the soft inflammatory tissue cannot be sutured safely and securely [3]. In the past completion pancreatectomy was preferred due to the fact that the complete source of necrosis and sepsis could be removed. However, completion pancreatectomy is technically very demanding, it requires splenectomy in most cases, and sometimes even total gastrectomy [1]. Another disadvantage is endocrine insufficiency. Moreover, the mortality of this procedure was inadequately high, reaching up to 100% [64]. Most authors nowadays prefer surgical peripancreatic drainage which a safer alternative. It is technically less demanding, the endocrine function of the pancreatic parenchyma is maintained and further surgical intervention is not required in most cases [66]. Completion pancreatectomy should no longer be considered a method of choice [1].

In distal pancreatectomy the PF is usually less severe, although it can be long-lasting. Several studies showed that endoscopic stent placement into the main pancreatic duct may resolve refractory grade C PF.

7. Economic Consequences of the PF

Pancreatic fistula has been proved to prolong the hospital stay and to increase the cost of treatment; these increases are progressively greater with increasing fistula severity [8]. In order to evaluate the cost of the treatment for various PF grades, a cost increase index (CII) can be determined. The CII for PF grades A, B, and C is calculated as multiples of the total cost for the no-fistula group. We validated the CII on own group of patients with pancreatic resection (unpublished data). The CII for PF grade A was 0.94, 1.66 for PF grade B, and 6.22 for PF grade C. It means that PF grade A has no further consequences and the cost of the treatment is similar to the group of patients with no PF. PF grade B slightly increases the cost of the treatment. PF grade C pronouncedly increases the cost of the treatment.

Several other studies analyzed the cost of pancreatic fistula treatment. A study by Holbrook included 30 patients who underwent pancreaticoduodenectomy. The authors reported that hospital costs increased by 76% due to postoperative complications. However, they did not analyze increases in cost specifically due to pancreatic fistula [67]. Another study, by Rodriguez included 66 patients who underwent distal pancreatectomy [68]. Pancreatic fistula was defined as a daily output of at least 30 ml of amylase-rich fluid (three times the serum concentration) from the surgically placed drain after postoperative day 5. Other pancreatic leak–related complications included a sterile collection, an abscess, and wound disruption. According to the ISGPF definition of PF, those complications would also be considered as PF. Furthermore the authors did not distinguish between transient and clinically relevant fistulas. Overall, 22 patients (33%) had complications attributed to pancreatic leak. The cost increase index (CII) in the pancreatic fistula group was double that of the non-fistula group. The average hospital stay was 5.2 ± 1.7 days for the no-fistula group and 16.6 ± 14.6 days for the fistula group. The main disadvantage of this study was that it did not use the ISGPF definition.

Pratt analyzed 256 consecutive pancreatic resections and compared the differences between pancreaticoduodenectomy, distal pancreatectomy, and central resections [8]. The authors used the ISGPF definition of fistula and found that the overall pancreatic fistula rate was 32.4%. The pancreatic fistula rates after pancreaticoduodenectomy and distal pancreatectomy were similar: 30% and 33%, respectively. The pancreatic fistula rate after central pancreatectomy in six patients reached 100%. In accordance with the results of Sauvanet [9], the fistulas that occurred after distal resections were more often biochemical and had no clinical consequences. The CII escalated after pancreaticoduodenectomy: 0.94, 1.45, and 7.09 for grade A, B, and C fistulas, respectively. However, the CII after distal pancreatectomy was 0.97, 2.27, and 2.53 for grade A, B, and C fistulas, respectively. Thus, the hospital costs were similar between grade B and C fistulas after distal pancreatectomy. The authors claimed that the impacts of grade B and C fistula after distal pancreatectomy are equivalent. However, only three patients had grade C fistula after distal pancreatectomy; this small number could have led to a bias in the results. Recently, a large study reported the results of 755 patients who underwent pancreaticoduodenectomy over a period of 10 years [26]. The overall pancreatic fistula rate was 19.5%, and the authors reported higher hospital costs for clinically significant pancreatic fistula. The CII for grade A, B, and C fistulas were 1.21, 2.66, and 6.16, respectively.

All the above-mentioned studies showed similar results of increase of the cost of the treatment with increase of the PF severity, and therefore the CII can be used universally in all pancreatic surgery centers regardless of the respective health care systems.

8. Delayed Hemorrhage and Other Consequences of PF

Delayed postoperative hemorrhage after pancreatic resection still represents an important source of concern. Standardized definition and classification had been lacking until recently. The International Study Group of Pancreatic Surgery proposed a new classification of postoperative hemorrhage based on time of onset, location, and severity of hemorrhage [69]. Early hemorrhage within 24 hours postoperatively is usually caused by technical failure of appropriate hemostasis at anastomotic sites, suture lines, or resections margins. Delayed hemorrhage is related to ulceration of anastomosis, leakage of venous anastomosis after portal vein resection, or erosion of peripancreatic vessels. Stepwise destruction of the vessel wall promotes the formation of pseudoaneurysms of the superior mesenteric artery and hepatic artery. Early identification of bleeding sites is difficult because of lack of specific symptoms. Repeated episodes of intraluminal bleeding or a decrease of hemoglobin are recognized as a “sentinel bleeding”. It may precede major hemorrhage from pseudoaneurysms, thus preventive measures must be taken. Contrast enhanced CT scan followed by interventional angiography provides accurate diagnosis and treatment in most cases. Postpancreatectomy hemorrhage is associated with PF in the majority of the cases. It usually occurs 13 to 27 days after the pancreatic resection. Delayed hemorrhage is not a frequent complication; its incidence is reported 3 to 5% [70]. However, it is a severe complication with lethality reaching around 30%.

Unlike early bleeding, which can be treated rather easily by urgent relaparotomy, delayed hemorrhage is more difficult to manage. Important factors which establish the diagnostic and therapeutic algorithms are: 1/ time of onset, 2/ severity of bleeding, 3/ intraluminal or extraluminal manifestation, 4/ underlying disease, 5/ type of index operation, and 6/ possible erosion of vascular structures due to PF [71]. The therapeutic options range from observation, monitoring, and fluid replacement to endoscopy, interventional angiography procedures and relaparotomy. Several suggested algorithms exist for the treatment of delayed postpancreatectomy hemorrhage [70, 71]. The method of choice in the first place is interventional angiography, which is successful in localizing and stopping the bleeding in the majority of cases. In some cases “blind” coiling of the gastroduodenal artery or the first two branches of the superior mesenteric artery can be performed without the site of bleeding being visualized [71]. Surgical exploration and hemostasis is recommended as a last option if previous methods of hemostasis have failed. It is because surgical access to the bleeding vessel is always difficult due to the pancreaticoenteric and bilioenteric anastomosis as well as the presence of postsurgical adhesions. The surgical procedure can encompass the following options: completion pancreatectomy, vascular reconstruction of the hepatic artery or superior mesenteric artery, and/or suture ligation of the bleeding site.

Another intraabdominal complication associated with PF is delayed gastric emptying (DFE). DGE is a persistent and frustrating complication after pancreaticoduodenectomy, with incidence varying from 12 to 42% [72]. It is more frequent after pylorus-saving procedure.

The wide range of results is due to the various definitions used. A new universal definition was published by the International Study Group on Pancreatic Surgery (ISGPS) in 2007 [72]. The pathogenesis of DGE remains controversial; it has been attributed to denervation and devascularization of the pylorus or to lower levels of cholecystokinin, secretin, and motilin. Several studies have shown a higher incidence of DGE in patients with PF.

PF was also considered a negative prognostic factor of survival in patients with pancreatic carcinoma. However, a recent large study with 1966 patients undergoing major pancreatic surgery did not support these findings [64]. According to Gebauer PF does not have a negative effect on the long-term survival of patients after pancreatic resection for malignancy.

9. Trauma of the Pancreas

Injuries to the pancreas are less common but may result in high morbidity and mortality. Pancreatic injury, vascular injury, and adjacent organ injuries often occur in combination. Pancreatic fistula is a source of complications in most cases. Injury to the pancreas is classified according to the AAST (American Association for the Surgery of Trauma) [Table 3]. Generally injuries are either blunt or penetrating.

The blunt injuries are caused by a wide range of mechanisms, e.g. traffic accidents, sport events injuries, etc. An important part of the injury mechanism is a compression of a subject towards the vertebral column, e.g. impact towards a steering wheel in a car accident or impact of handlebars towards the abdomen in a bicycle or motorcycle accidents [73].

The diagnostic process is more complicated in blunt injury. Contrast enhanced CT scan of the abdomen could show a laceration of the pancreas, but the specificity and sensitivity of this examination is rather low. Another option is the examination of serum amylase concentration. This, however, can be negative within 3 hours after the injury and thus it should be repeated. If the suspicion for pancreatic injury persists, endoscopic retrograde pancreatography (ERP) is recommended. It is more accurate than a CT scan; it can show the injury to the main pancreatic duct or pancreatic parenchyma.

Table 3. AAST classification of pancreatic trauma

I	Haematoma	Minor contusion without ductal injury
	Laceration	Superficial laceration without ductal injury
II	Haematoma	Major contusion without ductal injury or tissue loss
	Laceration	Major laceration without ductal injury or tissue loss
III	Laceration	Distal transection or pancreatic parenchymal injury with ductal injury
IV	Laceration	Proximal transection or pancreatic parenchymal injury involving the ampulla
V	Laceration	Massive disruption of the pancreatic head

It is also a therapeutical modality because a stent into the main pancreatic duct may be inserted. Another diagnostic option in stable patients with pancreatic duct injury is magnetic resonance pancreatography (MRP). However, the experience with MRP in these cases is not great. Furthermore, it is a rather time-consuming examination [74].

Penetrating abdominal injuries are more frequent in countries with higher levels of criminality and with better availability of shotguns. All patients with shotgun injuries to the abdomen are indicated for surgical exploration of the abdomen, with the pancreatic injury often discovered during the exploration. On the other hand, blunt trauma of the pancreas is more frequently diagnosed using the above mentioned methods and conservative treatment is more often advocated [75].

There are more options for treating pancreatic injury. Pancreatic injury of grades I and II are best treated using a conservative approach or simple drainage. Minor laceration of the pancreatic capsule can be treated with suture and/or omentoplasty. Some authors recommend administration of octreotide to decrease the PF rate as in elective pancreatic resections. If a symptomatic pseudocyst evolves, it can be treated with endoscopic pseudocystogastrostomy or percutaneous external drainage [76].

Patients with grade III pancreatic injury are usually treated with distal pancreatectomy. Patients with grade III or IV pancreatic injury can be treated with a suture of the excluded jejunal loop to the lacerated part of pancreas. Patients with injury grades IV and V can be treated by a simple drainage or pancreaticoduodenectomy [77]. However, pancreaticoduodenectomy is a formidable procedure and it is performed only exceptionally for complex pancreatic and duodenal injuries. The indications include massive uncontrolled bleeding from the pancreatic head and adjacent vascular structures, and non-reconstructable injury of the pancreatic head, duodenum or distal common bile duct when primary repair is not feasible. The resection can be performed without reconstruction as part of the damage control surgery, and the reconstruction is then performed within 48 hours after stabilization of the patient. This procedure carries a high morbidity (up to 80%) and high mortality (up to 30%) [77].

Injury to the pancreas can also occur iatrogenically in surgical procedures on adjacent organs, e.g. splenectomy, gastrectomy, colectomy, left radical nephrectomy, left adrenalectomy, or vascular surgery (abdominal aorta repair), etc. Pancreatic injury and subsequent PF is a possible complication due to the close anatomical vicinity of the pancreas. The anatomical situation may be altered in inflammatory diseases of the resected organs or locally advanced tumors. PF in these cases is usually less severe (Grade A), does not require any additional treatment besides keeping the preoperatively placed drains for a longer period of time and resolves spontaneously within 3 weeks; however it can prolong the postoperative course.

Conclusion

Pancreatic fistula is a common complication after pancreatic resections. This complication is not life-threatening in most cases but it prolongs the hospital stay, increases the cost of the treatment and delays adjuvant treatment in malignant disease. It is advisable to use a universal definition in order to compare results of various surgical techniques or interventions, and results among centers or individual surgeons. The definition of PF according to the ISGPF has been validated in several studies and is widely accepted. Most of the risk factors of developing PF cannot be influenced. There are basically only two possible options to lower the rates of PF: pharmacological interventions and technical modifications of the pancreatic remnant management. There is no consensus on which surgical technique is optimal; the skill of the operating surgeon, the individual experience, the experience of the center, and the volume of the center may be even more important than the technique used. The diagnosis of PF must be prompt in order to minimize possibly devastating effects. PF is associated with other intra-abdominal complications such as delayed hemorrhage or delayed gastric emptying. PF therapy consists of conservative measures in majority of cases. Reoperation is advocated only in the most severe cases of PF and, if reoperation must be performed, simple surgical peripancreatic drainage is preferred over completion pancreatectomy.

REFERENCES

[1] Buchler MW; Wagner M; Schmied BM; Uhl W; Friess H; Z'Graggen K. Changes in morbidity after pancreatic resection: toward the end of completion pancreatectomy. *Arch. Surg.*, 2003. 138, 12: p. 1310-1314.

[2] DeOliveira ML; Winter JM; Schafer M; Cunningham SC; Cameron JL; Yeo CJ; Clavien PA. Assessment of complications after pancreatic surgery: A novel grading system applied to 633 patients undergoing pancreaticoduodenectomy. *Ann. Surg.*, 2006. 244, 6: p. 931-937.

[3] Callery MP; Pratt WB; Vollmer CM Jr. Prevention and management of pancreatic fistula. *J. Gastrointest. Surg.*, 2009. 13, 1: p. 163-173.

[4] Pratt WB; Maithel SK; Vanounou T; Huang ZS; Callery MP; Vollmer CM Jr. Clinical and economic validation of the International Study Group of Pancreatic Fistula (ISGPF) classification scheme. *Ann. Surg.*, 2007. 245, 3: p. 443-451.

[5] Bassi C; Dervenis C; Butturini G; Fingerhut A; Yeo C; Izbicki J; Neoptolemos J; Sarr M; Traverso W; Buchler M. Postoperative pancreatic fistula: an international study group (ISGPF) definition. *Surgery*, 2005. 138, 1: p. 8-13.

[6] Shrikhande SV; D'Souza MA. Pancreatic fistula after pancreatectomy: evolving definitions, preventive strategies and modern management. *World J. Gastroenterol.*, 2008. 14, 38: p. 5789-5796.

[7] Bassi C; Butturini G; Molinari E; Mascetta G; Salvia R; Falconi M; Gumbs A; Pederzoli P. Pancreatic fistula rate after pancreatic resection. The importance of definitions. *Dig. Surg.*, 2004. 21, 1: p. 54-59.

[8] Pratt W; Maithel SK; Vanounou T; Callery MP; Vollmer CM Jr. Postoperative pancreatic fistulas are not equivalent after proximal, distal, and central pancreatectomy. *J. Gastrointest. Surg.*, 2006. 10, 9: p. 1264-1278.

[9] Sauvanet A; Partensky C; Sastre B; Gigot JF; Fagniez PL; Tuech JJ; Millat B; Berdah S; Dousset B; Jaeck D; Le Treut YP; Letoublon C. Medial pancreatectomy: a multi-institutional retrospective study of 53 patients by the French Pancreas Club. *Surgery*, 2002. 132, 5: p. 836-843.

[10] Seth TN. The Activation of Pancreatic Juice by Enterokinase. *Biochem. J.*, 1924. 18, 6: p. 1401-1416.

[11] Lin, JW; Cameron JL; Yeo CJ; Riall TS; Lillemoe KD. Risk factors and outcomes in postpancreaticoduodenectomy pancreaticocutaneous fistula. *J. Gastrointest. Surg.*, 2004. 8, 8: p. 951-959.

[12] Yeo CJ; Cameron JL; Lillemoe KD; Sauter PK; Coleman J; Sohn TA; Campbell KA; Choti MA. Does prophylactic octreotide decrease the rates of pancreatic fistula and other complications after pancreaticoduodenectomy? Results of a prospective randomized placebo-controlled trial. *Ann. Surg.*, 2000. 232, 3: p. 419-429.

[13] Lai EC; Lau SH; Lau WY. Measures to prevent pancreatic fistula after pancreatoduodenectomy: a comprehensive review. *Arch. Surg.*, 2009. 144, 11: p. 1074-1080.

[14] Matsusue S; Takeda H; Nakamura Y; Nishimura S; Koizumi S. A prospective analysis of the factors influencing pancreaticojejunostomy performed using a single method, in 100 consecutive pancreaticoduodenectomies. *Surg. Today*, 1998. 28, 7: p. 719-726.

[15] Gaujoux, S; Cortes A; Couvelard A; Noullet S; Clavel L; Rebours V; Levy P; Sauvanet A; Ruszniewski P; Belghiti J. Fatty pancreas and increased body mass index are risk factors of pancreatic fistula after pancreaticoduodenectomy. *Surgery*, 2010. 148, 1: p. 15-23.

[16] Yeh TS; Jan YY; Jeng LB; Hwang TL; Wang CS; Chen SC; Chao TC; Chen MF. Pancreaticojejunal anastomotic leak after pancreaticoduodenectomy - multivariate analysis of perioperative risk factors. *J. Surg. Res.*, 1997. 67, 2: p. 119-125.

[17] Ban D; Shimada K; Konishi M; Saiura A; Hashimoto M; Uesaka K. Stapler and nonstapler closure of the pancreatic remnant after distal pancreatectomy: multicenter retrospective analysis of 388 patients. *World J. Surg.*, 2012. 36, 8: p. 1866-1873.

[18] Chu CK; Mazo AE; Sarmiento JM; Staley CA; Adsay NV; Umpierrez GE; Kooby DA. Impact of diabetes mellitus on perioperative outcomes after resection for pancreatic adenocarcinoma. *J. Am. Coll. Surg.*, 2010. 210, 4: p. 463-473.

[19] Subhedar PD; Patel SH; Kneuertz PJ; Maithel SK; Staley CA; Sarmiento JM; Galloway JR; Kooby DA. Risk factors for pancreatic fistula after stapled gland transection. *Am. Surg.*, 2011. 77, 8: p. 965-970.

[20] Cheng Q; Zhang B; Zhang Y; Jiang X; Zhang B; Yi B; Luo X; Wu M. Predictive factors for complications after pancreaticoduodenectomy. *J. Surg. Res.*, 2007. 139, 1: p. 22-29.

[21] Kleeff, J; Diener MK; Z'Graggen K; Hinz U; Wagner M; Bachmann J; Zehetner J; Muller MW; Friess H; Buchler MW. Distal pancreatectomy: risk factors for surgical failure in 302 consecutive cases. *Ann. Surg.*, 2007. 245, 4: p. 573-582.

[22] Cheng TY; Sheth K; White RR; Ueno T; Hung CF; Clary BM; Pappas TN; Tyler DS. Effect of neoadjuvant chemoradiation on operative mortality and morbidity for pancreaticoduodenectomy. *Ann. Surg. Oncol.*, 2006. 13, 1: p. 66-74.

[23] Schmidt, CM; Turrini O; Parikh P; House MG; Zyromski NJ; Nakeeb A; Howard TJ; Pitt HA; Lillemoe KD. Effect of hospital volume, surgeon experience, and surgeon volume on patient outcomes after pancreaticoduodenectomy: a single-institution experience. *Arch. Surg.*, 2010. 145, 7: p. 634-640.

[24] Gouma DJ; van Geenen RC; van Gulik TM; de Haan RJ; de Wit LT; Busch OR; Obertop H. Rates of complications and death after pancreaticoduodenectomy: risk factors and the impact of hospital volume. *Ann. Surg*., 2000. 232, 6: p. 786-795.

[25] Sosa JA; Bowman HM; Gordon TA; Bass EB; Yeo CJ; Lillemoe KD; Pitt HA; Tielsch JM; Cameron JL. Importance of hospital volume in the overall management of pancreatic cancer. *Ann. Surg*., 1998. 228, 3: p. 429-438.

[26] Daskalaki D; Butturini G; Molinari E; Crippa S; Pederzoli P; Bassi C. A grading system can predict clinical and economic outcomes of pancreatic fistula after pancreaticoduodenectomy: results in 755 consecutive patients. *Langenbecks Arch. Surg*., 2011. 396, 1: p. 91-98.

[27] Klempa I; Schwedes U; Usadel KH. Prevention of postoperative pancreatic complications following duodenopancreatectomy using somatostatin. *Chirurg*, 1979. 50, 7: p. 427-431.

[28] Raptis S; Schlegel W; Lehmann E; Dollinger HC; Zoupas C. Effects of somatostatin on the exocrine pancreas and the release of duodenal hormones. *Metabolism*, 1978. 27, 9 Suppl 1: p. 1321-1328.

[29] Lamberts SW; van der Lely AJ; de Herder WW; Hofland LJ. Octreotide. *N. Engl. J. Med*., 1996. 334, 4: p. 246-254.

[30] Falconi M; Contro C; Ballabio M ;Bassi C; Salvia R; Pederzoli P, Evaluation of lanreotide effects on human exocrine pancreatic secretion after a single dose: preliminary study. *Dig. Liver Dis*., 2002. 34, 2: p. 127-132.

[31] Ritz MA; Drewe J; Ziel A; Hildebrand P; Schneider P; Lahlou N; Beglinger C. The effects of vapreotide, a somatostatin analogue, on gastric acidity, gallbladder emptying and hormone release after 1 week of continuous subcutaneous infusion in normal subjects. *Br. J. Clin. Pharmacol*., 1999. 47, 2: p. 195-201.

[32] Buchler M; Friess H; Klempa I; Hermanek P; Sulkowski U; Becker H; Schafmayer A; Baca I; Lorenz D; Meister R et al. Role of octreotide in the prevention of postoperative complications following pancreatic resection. *Am. J. Surg*., 1992. 163, 1: p. 125-130.

[33] Friess H; Beger HG; Sulkowski U; Becker H; Hofbauer B; Dennler HJ; Buchler MW. Randomized controlled multicentre study of the prevention of complications by octreotide in patients undergoing surgery for chronic pancreatitis. *Br. J. Surg*., 1995. 82, 9: p. 1270-1273.

[34] Montorsi M; Zago M; Mosca F; Capussotti L; Zotti E; Ribotta G; Fegiz G; Fissi S; Roviaro G; Peracchia A et al. Efficacy of octreotide in the prevention of pancreatic fistula after elective pancreatic resections: a prospective, controlled, randomized clinical trial. *Surgery*, 1995. 117, 1: p. 26-31.

[35] Pederzoli P; Bassi C; Falconi M; Camboni MG. Efficacy of octreotide in the prevention of complications of elective pancreatic surgery. Italian Study Group. *Br. J. Surg*., 1994. 81, 2: p. 265-269.

[36] Lowy AM; Lee JE; Pisters PW; Davidson BS; Fenoglio CJ; Stanford P; Jinnah R; Evans DB. Prospective, randomized trial of octreotide to prevent pancreatic fistula after pancreaticoduodenectomy for malignant disease. *Ann. Surg*., 1997. 226, 5: p. 632-641.

[37] Suc B; Msika S; Piccinini M; Fourtanier G; Hay JM; Flamant Y; Fingerhut A; Fagniez PL; Chipponi J. Octreotide in the prevention of intra-abdominal complications following elective pancreatic resection: a prospective, multicenter randomized controlled trial. *Arch. Surg*., 2004. 139, 3: p. 288-294.

[38] Gouillat C; Chipponi J; Baulieux J; Partensky C; Saric J; Gayet B. Randomized controlled multicentre trial of somatostatin infusion after pancreaticoduodenectomy. *Br. J. Surg.*, 2001. 88, 11: p. 1456-1462.

[39] Shan YS; Sy ED; Lin PW. Role of somatostatin in the prevention of pancreatic stump-related morbidity following elective pancreaticoduodenectomy in high-risk patients and elimination of surgeon-related factors: prospective, randomized, controlled trial. *World J. Surg.*, 2003. 27, 6: p. 709-714.

[40] Londong W; Angerer M; Kutz K; Landgraf R; Londong V. Diminishing efficacy of octreotide (SMS 201-995) on gastric functions of healthy subjects during one-week administration. *Gastroenterology*, 1989. 96, 3: p. 713-722.

[41] Closset J; Journe S; Mboti F; El Nakadi I; Gelin M. Randomized controlled trial comparing somatostatin with octreotide in the prevention of complications after pancreatectomy. *Hepatogastroenterology*, 2008. 55, 86-87: p. 1818-1823.

[42] Sarr MG. The potent somatostatin analogue vapreotide does not decrease pancreas-specific complications after elective pancreatectomy: a prospective, multicenter, double-blinded, randomized, placebo-controlled trial. *J. Am. Coll. Surg.*, 2003. 196, 4: p. 556-564.

[43] Čečka F; Jon B; Šubrt Z; Ferko A. The effect of somatostatin and its analogs in the prevention of pancreatic fistula after elective pancreatic surgery. *Eur. Surg.*, 2012. 44, 2: p. 99-108.

[44] Pitt SC; Pitt HA; Baker MS; Christians K; Touzios JG; Kiely JM; Weber SM; Wilson SD; Howard TJ; Talamonti MS; Rikkers LF. Small pancreatic and periampullary neuroendocrine tumors: resect or enucleate? *J. Gastrointest. Surg.*, 2009. 13, 9: p. 1692-1698.

[45] Brient C; Regenet N; Sulpice L; Brunaud L; Mucci-Hennekine S; Carrere N; Milin J; Ayav A; Pradere B; Hamy A; Bresler L; Meunier B; Mirallie E. Risk factors for postoperative pancreatic fistulization subsequent to enucleation. *J. Gastrointest. Surg.*, 2012. 16, 10: p. 1883-1887.

[46] Brown KM; Shoup M; Abodeely A; Hodul P; Brems JJ; Aranha GV. Central pancreatectomy for benign pancreatic lesions. *HPB* (Oxford), 2006. 8, 2: p. 142-147.

[47] Shrikhande SV; Qureshi SS; Rajneesh N; Shukla PJ. Pancreatic anastomoses after pancreaticoduodenectomy: do we need further studies? *World J. Surg.*, 2005. 29, 12: p. 1642-1649.

[48] Wente MN; Shrikhande SV; Muller MW; Diener MK; Seiler CM; Friess H; Buchler MW. Pancreaticojejunostomy versus pancreaticogastrostomy: systematic review and meta-analysis. *Am. J. Surg.*, 2007. 193, 2: p. 171-183.

[49] Bassi C; Falconi M; Molinari E; Mantovani W; Butturini G; Gumbs AA; Salvia R; Pederzoli P. Duct-to-mucosa versus end-to-side pancreaticojejunostomy reconstruction after pancreaticoduodenectomy: results of a prospective randomized trial. *Surgery*, 2003. 134, 5: p. 766-771.

[50] Berger AC; Howard TJ; Kennedy EP; Sauter PK; Bower-Cherry M; Dutkevitch S; Hyslop T; Schmidt CM; Rosato EL; Lavu H; Nakeeb A; Pitt HA; Lillemoe KD; Yeo CJ. Does type of pancreaticojejunostomy after pancreaticoduodenectomy decrease rate of pancreatic fistula? A randomized, prospective, dual-institution trial. *J. Am. Coll. Surg.*, 2009. 208, 5: p. 738-747.

[51] Chou FF; Sheen-Chen SM; Chen YS; Chen MC; Chen CL. Postoperative morbidity and mortality of pancreaticoduodenectomy for periampullary cancer. *Eur. J. Surg.*, 1996. 162, 6: p. 477-481.

[52] Tran KT; Smeenk HG; van Eijck CH; Kazemier G; Hop WC; Greve JW; Terpstra OT; Zijlstra JA; Klinkert P; Jeekel H. Pylorus preserving pancreaticoduodenectomy versus standard Whipple procedure: a prospective, randomized, multicenter analysis of 170 patients with pancreatic and periampullary tumors. *Ann. Surg.*, 2004. 240, 5: p. 738-745.

[53] Poon RT; Fan ST; Lo CM; Ng KK; Yuen WK; Yeung C; Wong J. External drainage of pancreatic duct with a stent to reduce leakage rate of pancreaticojejunostomy after pancreaticoduodenectomy: a prospective randomized trial. *Ann. Surg.*, 2007. 246, 3: p. 425-433.

[54] Winter JM; Cameron JL; Campbell KA; Chang DC; Riall TS; Schulick RD; Choti MA; Coleman J; Hodgin MB; Sauter PK; Sonnenday CJ; Wolfgang CL; Marohn MR; Yeo CJ. Does pancreatic duct stenting decrease the rate of pancreatic fistula following pancreaticoduodenectomy? Results of a prospective randomized trial. *J. Gastrointest. Surg.*, 2006. 10, 9: p. 1280-1290.

[55] Wada K, Traverso LW. Pancreatic anastomotic leak after the Whipple procedure is reduced using the surgical microscope. *Surgery*, 2006. 139, 6: p. 735-742.

[56] Nathan H; Cameron JL; Goodwin CR; Seth AK; Edil BH; Wolfgang CL; Pawlik TM; Schulick RD; Choti MA. Risk factors for pancreatic leak after distal pancreatectomy. *Ann. Surg.*, 2009. 250, 2: p. 277-281.

[57] Reeh M; Nentwich MF; Bogoevski D; Koenig AM; Gebauer F; Tachezy M; Izbicki JR; Bockhorn M. High surgical morbidity following distal pancreatectomy: still an unsolved problem. *World J. Surg.*, 2011. 35, 5: p. 1110-1117.

[58] Ferrone CR; Warshaw AL; Rattner DW; Berger D; Zheng H; Rawal B; Rodriguez R; Thayer SP; Fernandez-del Castillo C. Pancreatic fistula rates after 462 distal pancreatectomies: staplers do not decrease fistula rates. *J. Gastrointest. Surg.*, 2008. 12, 10: p. 1691-1697.

[59] Diener MK; Seiler CM; Rossion I; Kleeff J; Glanemann M; Butturini G; Tomazic A; Bruns CJ; Busch OR; Farkas S; Belyaev O; Neoptolemos JP; Halloran C; Keck T; Niedergethmann M; Gellert K; Witzigmann H; Kollmar O; Langer P; Steger U; Neudecker J; Berrevoet F; Ganzera S; Heiss MM; Luntz SP; Bruckner T; Kieser M; Buchler MW. Efficacy of stapler versus hand-sewn closure after distal pancreatectomy (DISPACT): a randomised, controlled multicentre trial. *Lancet*, 2011. 377, 9776: p. 1514-1522.

[60] Jusoh AC; Ammori BJ. Laparoscopic versus open distal pancreatectomy: a systematic review of comparative studies. *Surg. Endosc.*, 2012. 26, 4: p. 904-913.

[61] Nigri GR; Rosman AS; Petrucciani N; Fancellu A; Pisano M; Zorcolo L; Ramacciato G; Melis M. Metaanalysis of trials comparing minimally invasive and open distal pancreatectomies. *Surg. Endosc.*, 2011. 25, 5: p. 1642-1651.

[62] Song KB; Kim SC; Park JB; Kim YH ;Jung YS; Kim MH; Lee SK; Seo DW; Lee SS; Park do II; Han DJ. Single-center experience of laparoscopic left pancreatic resection in 359 consecutive patients: changing the surgical paradigm of left pancreatic resection. *Surg. Endosc.*, 2011. 25, 10: p. 3364-3372.

[63] Sepesi B; Moalem J; Galka E; Salzman P; Schoeniger LO. The Influence of Staple Size on Fistula Formation Following Distal Pancreatectomy. *J. Gastrointest. Surg*., 2012. 16, 2: p. 267-274.

[64] Gebauer F; Kloth K; Tachezy M; Vashist YK; Cataldegirmen G; Izbicki JR; Bockhorn M. Options and limitations in applying the fistula classification by the International Study Group for Pancreatic Fistula. *Ann. Surg*., 2012. 256, 1: p. 130-138.

[65] Kleespies A; Albertsmeier M; Obeidat F; Seeliger H; Jauch KW; Bruns CJ. The challenge of pancreatic anastomosis. *Langenbecks Arch. Surg*., 2008. 393, 4: p. 459-471.

[66] Haddad LB; Scatton O; Randone B; Andraus W; Massault PP; Dousset B; Soubrane O. Pancreatic fistula after pancreaticoduodenectomy: the conservative treatment of choice. *HPB* (Oxford), 2009. 11, 3: p. 203-209.

[67] Holbrook RF; Hargrave K; Traverso LW. A prospective cost analysis of pancreatoduodenectomy. *Am. J. Surg*., 1996. 171, 5: p. 508-511.

[68] Rodriguez JR; Germes SS; Pandharipande PV; Gazelle GS; Thayer SP; Warshaw AL; Fernandez-del Castillo C. Implications and cost of pancreatic leak following distal pancreatic resection. *Arch. Surg*., 2006. 141, 4: p. 361-365.

[69] Wente MN; Veit JA; Bassi C; Dervenis C; Fingerhut A; Gouma DJ; Izbicki JR; Neoptolemos JP; Padbury RT; Sarr MG; Yeo CJ; Buchler MW. Postpancreatectomy hemorrhage (PPH): an International Study Group of Pancreatic Surgery (ISGPS) definition. *Surgery*, 2007. 142, 1: p. 20-25.

[70] Roulin D; Cerantola Y; Demartines N; Schafer M. Systematic review of delayed postoperative hemorrhage after pancreatic resection. *J. Gastrointest. Surg*., 2011. 15, 6: p. 1055-1062.

[71] Yekebas EF; Wolfram L; Cataldegirmen G; Habermann CR; Bogoevski D; Koenig AM; Kaifi J; Schurr PG; Bubenheim M; Nolte-Ernsting C; Adam G; Izbicki JR. Postpancreatectomy hemorrhage: diagnosis and treatment: an analysis in 1669 consecutive pancreatic resections. *Ann. Surg*., 2007. 246, 2: p. 269-280.

[72] Wente MN; Bassi C; Dervenis C; Fingerhut A ; Gouma DJ; Izbicki JR; Neoptolemos JP; Padbury RT; Sarr MG; Traverso LW; Yeo CJ; Buchler MW. Delayed gastric emptying (DGE) after pancreatic surgery: a suggested definition by the International Study Group of Pancreatic Surgery (ISGPS). *Surgery*, 2007. 142, 5: p. 761-768.

[73] Pata G; Casella C; Di Betta E; Grazioli L; Salerni B. Extension of nonoperative management of blunt pancreatic trauma to include grade III injuries: a safety analysis. *World J. Surg*., 2009. 33, 8: p. 1611-1617.

[74] Subramanian A; Dente CJ; Feliciano DV. The management of pancreatic trauma in the modern era. *Surg. Clin. North Am*., 2007. 87, 6: p. 1515-1532, x.

[75] Asensio JA; Petrone P; Roldan G; Pakart R; Salim A. Pancreatic and duodenal injuries. Complex and lethal. *Scand. J. Surg*., 2002. 91, 1: p. 81-86.

[76] Chinnery GE; Madiba TE. Pancreaticoduodenal injuries: re-evaluating current management approaches. *S. Afr. J. Surg*., 2010. 48, 1: p. 10-14.

[77] Asensio JA; Petrone P; Roldan G; Kuncir E; Demetriades D. Pancreaticoduodenectomy: a rare procedure for the management of complex pancreaticoduodenal injuries. *J. Am. Coll. Surg*., 2003. 197, 6: p. 937-942.

In: Fistuals and Fissures
Editors: Dmitri Pavlovich and Sergei Ivanovich

ISBN: 978-1-62618-068-0

Chapter 2

CUTANEOUS ADVANCEMENT FLAP COMBINED WITH "TAILORED" LATERAL INTERNAL SPHINCTEROTOMY FOR CHRONIC ANAL FISSURE: RESULTS FROM OUR PROSPECTIVE DATABASE AND REVIEW OF THE LITERATURE

George E. Theodoropoulos*
Colorectal Unit, First Department of Propaedeutic Surgery, Athens Medical School, Athens, Greece

ABSTRACT

Lateral internal sphincterotomy (LIS) is considered the surgical treatment of choice for chronic idiopathic anal fissure. Except for minor episodes of impaired continence, LIS routinely does not include wound closure, which may lead to complications of secondary wound healing (anal stenosis, keyhole deformity). Flap techniques have the advantage of the primary wound healing avoiding scar formation as a risk for minor anal incontinence. Primary wound healing after fissurectomy is usually impossible owing to increased tension on the suture lines and can only be achieved by a tension-free skin graft. Although no difference has been proven between the two techniques, a lack of data exists on the results of a combined procedure.

Over a period of 3 years, 45 patients who underwent LIS + dermal flap were recruited and prospectively followed-up for a minimum of 6 months. Following a "tailored" LIS (internal sphincter division "up to the level of the fissure apex" a fissurectomy was undertaken. The hypertrophic papilla when present was excised, and the sides of the fissure were freshened by sharp scalpel dissection. A modified, trapezoid-like Y-V flap, consisted of skin and subcutaneous fat, was dissected free of the fibers of the subcutaneous external anal sphincter to allow tension-free advancement into the fissure base. The advanced flap was sutured to the site of the previous fissure.

* Corresponding author: George E. Theodoropoulos, MD, PhD, FACS. Ass Professor of Surgery, Athens Medical School, Address: 7 Semitelou Street, GR-11528 Athens, Greece. Tel: +30 6945463593; Fax: +30 2107707574; E-mail: georgetheocrs@live.com.

All except one patient healed completely within 30 days from operation. The intensity of pain post-defecation was reduced significantly compared to the preoperative values even from the first defecation ($p<0.0001$). None of the patients complained of pain at the end of the first postoperative week. Analgesics were not required beyond the 3rd POD. Episodes of minor bleeding occurred in 8 patients in during the period of the first 2 weeks. The only remarkable complication recorded postoperatively was a partial break down occurred in one case, which was managed conservatively. At the 6 months follow-up appointment, no recurrences were recorded and in no case was further surgery necessary. After a median follow-up of 20 months (range 8-36), when all patients were contacted by phone, no patient reported pain or clinical symptoms of anal fissure.

Review of the literature and current results support that flap techniques have the advantage of primary wound healing avoiding scar formation as a risk for minor anal incontinence. The addition of a dermal flap after LIS results in excellent healing and minimal postoperative discomfort. Even though it extends the operative time, at our academic clinical practice, we have completely changed our therapeutic strategy, incorporating the flap in all cases of surgically treated fissures.

INTRODUCTION

The principal aim of treatment for chronic idiopathic anal fissures is to decrease internal sphincter tone and hence increase the blood flow with subsequent tissue healing [1-5]. The technique of lateral internal sphincterotomy (LIS) is considered the treatment of choice and to date remains the standard [6-9]. Conventional LIS which includes division of internal sphincter up to the level of the dentate line may suffer as a technique due to the minor episodes of impaired postoperative continence [10-13]. Limiting the height of the sphincterotomy to the length of the fissure in order to create a more controlled "tailored" LIS may partially overcome continence disturbances [14-16].

LIS routinely does not include wound closure, which may lead to complications of secondary wound healing, such as anal stenosis and keyhole deformity. In an effort to improve and fasten fissure healing and to achieve fissure revision, the fissurectomy has been proposed, which involves freshening of the anal fissure, excision of the fissure edges, curetting or excision of the fissure base and possibly excision of sentinel skin tags and anal polyps [17-20]. Such an excision, though, may lead to a wide bare anal area, which may still require a long healing period. On the other hand, by solely applying LIS for management of an anal fissure may alleviate patients' discomfort due to the inherent sphincter hypertonicity, but may not be directly efficient on the component of pain related to the presence of a gaping region and an exposed internal anal sphincter at the fissure site. Finally, secondary wound healing with scar formation after LIS or plain fissurectomy may contribute to the unavoidable risk for minor anal incontinence.

Flap anoplasty procedures have been widely used in the treatment of chronic anal fissures [21-42]. These procedures involve fashioning a local flap to cover the fissure defect. As flap procedures do not involve disruption of the internal anal sphincter, they are particularly useful in patients with normal anal pressures or in fissures secondary to obstetric trauma where there is often associated internal sphincter disruption [22, 23, 30, 31, 34]. Although flap anoplasty procedures have a defined role in treatment of fissures in such clinical circumstances, their role in cases with raised anal pressures has been examined, but not clearly defined and incorporated in the routine clinical practice [21, 24, 37, 40, 41]. Flap techniques have also the advantage of the primary wound healing with limitation or even elimination of scar in the previous fissure position. Moreover, primary wound healing after fissurectomy is usually impossible owing to increased tension on the suture lines and can only be achieved by a tension-free skin graft. No difference at healing rates has been proven between LIS and flap anoplasty, when applied as isolated procedures [24, 37, 40]. Up to recently, a lack of data had been existing on the results of a combined procedure. At the time of this writing, though, the results of a randomized study between LIS, advancement flap and "tailored" LIS combined with a flap were reported, which substantiated a significant clinical advantage on the combined procedure for the surgical treatment of anal fissure [41].

Patients and Methods

Patient Identification and Data Collection

Prospectively collected data of 45 consecutive patients undergoing LIS and dermal flap for symptomatic chronic anal fissure from January 2009 until January 2012 was used. In 2009, we modified the surgical technique for treatment of chronic anal fissure in order to explore the efficacy and potential advantages of the addition of a dermal flap to a more conservative "tailored" LIS for purposes of primary wound healing and minimization of minor incontinence associated with the previously "conventional" sphincterotomy, which was routinely applied in our surgical practice. When suspicion existed for increased likelihood of postoperative impaired continence, such as in females with "weak" sphincters, the sphincterotomy was not applied at all. Such a scenario has occurred in 5 female patients and those cases were not included in the current analysis. Data collection for all patients undergoing LIS and dermal flap included preoperative symptoms and pathological findings of the anus, fissure position, length of hospital stay, clinical course, and postoperative follow-up (Table 1). Data for analysis were tabulated from an inpatient computerized database. Written informed consent was obtained from all patients before surgery. Exclusion criteria were the presence of anal abscess, anal fistula, stenosis, and any associated conditions, such as inflammatory bowel disease, malignancy, documented specific infection. Chronic anal fissure was defined as the presence of a fibrous induration, sentinel pile, hypertrophied anal papillae, or exposed internal sphincter fibers. All patients presented with a chronic anal fissure refractory to well-practiced topical medical therapy and conservative management with high fiber dietary supplementation, analgesics, and warm sitz baths for more than 2 months. The failure of such measures and the patient's desire for surgical treatment led to application of the combined "LIS and dermal flap" technique. Primary endpoints of the study was the degree of postoperative pain at distinct time-points [1st, 7th, 15th postoperative day (POD), at the 1st defecation, defecation at the 7th and 15th day] and the healing rate at the fixed postoperative assessment appointments. Secondary endpoints included episodes of minor incontinence, postoperative complications, re-operations, satisfaction rate and any further symptoms and concerns from the patients' perspective. To achieve these goals, all patients were subjected to a strict follow-up appointment schedule at the end of the 1st and 2nd weeks, the 1st, 3rd and 6th month. Independently of these scheduled appointments, patients were seen on request. Telephone interviews were also conducted with all patients at the end of the follow-up period (July 2012).

Table 1. Patients' characteristics, symptoms and preoperative anal examination results

Results	LIS + Flap
N	45
Age (years), mean; SD; range	40, 12.5; 23–67
Gender (female/male)	13/32
Fissure location Posterior midline, n (%) Posterior and anterior midline, n(%)	 43 (95.5) 2 (4.4)
Skin tag, n (%)	39 (86.6)
Anal polyp, n (%)	30 (66.6)
Symptoms preoperatively Pain, n (%) Minor bleeding, n (%) Itching, n (%) Constipation, n (%)	 45 (100) 35 (77.7) 1 (2.2) 21 (46.6)

Operative Technique

"LIS and dermal flap" were performed as an inpatient surgical procedure. All patients were treated by the same colorectal surgeon (G.T.). Before surgery, all patients received a small volume of phosphate saline enema. Metronidazole (Flagyl, Sanofi-Aventis Inc, Athens, Greece) was administered intravenously in a dose of 500 mg during induction of anesthesia. Subsequently, the same dose was administered iv twice every 8 hours and then it was prescribed per os for 5 more days 3 times daily. The majority of procedures were performed under general anesthesia with the patient at a lithotomy position with the thighs hyperflexed. A Foley catheter was not used. To enhance postoperative pain control and to facilitate sphincteric muscle relaxation, a posterior nerve block with local infiltration of a long-acting anesthetic (Ropivacaine; Naropeine 0.2%, Cana Inc, Athens, Greece) or just Xylocaine 2% was performed. Epinephrine was not contained in either solution for fear of compromising the blood supply. The solution was injected subcutaneously along the anal verges in the 4 quadrants (20 mL) and deep into the 2 ischiorectal fossae (10-20 mL).

LIS Technique

A bivalve Pratt anal speculum was gently inserted into the anal canal, taking care to avoid uncontrolled sphincter dilation. The intersphincteric groove was identified at 3 o'clock. After skin incision, the internal anal sphincter was identified, elevated with the passage of a Pean forceps into the intersphincteric groove and divided with diathermy under direct vision and "up to the level of the fissure apex", in order to complete a "tailored" LIS. The incision was then primarily closed with a continuous 4/0 Vicryl suture (Ethicon Inc, USA).

Dermal Flap Technique

A fissurectomy was undertaken in all cases. The hypertrophic papilla when present was excised and the sides of the fissure were freshened by sharp scalpel dissection. The base of the fissure was gently de-epithelialized, and granulation tissue was carefully curetted to leave a clean exposed internal anal sphincter. A decision was then made as to whether part of the distal skin tag was of sufficient quality to be used as the cephalad portion of the flap, or whether it was fibrotic and poorly vascularized, in which case it was excised. Longitudinal incisions were then performed along both sides posterior to the wound using a scalpel (Figure 1). A tension-free modified, trapezoid-like flap, consisted of skin and subcutaneous fat was then raised. To ensure a broad-based flap with ideal blood supply, the length of the flap was at least 1.5 times the length of the fissure. The dermal flap was dissected free of the fibers of the posterior aspect of the internal sphincter and the subcutaneous portion of the external anal sphincter to allow tension-free advancement into the fissure base. The advanced flap was sutured to the adjacent anal mucosa at its apex, anoderm at its sides, and perineal skin at the anal margin, with interrupted absorbable 3/0 Vicryl (Ethicon Inc, USA) (Figure 1). Electrocautery was avoided during flap dissection and minor bleeding usually stopped after the flap was sutured to the anal canal. This technique allowed primary closure of the entire wound area. Operation time ranged from 30 to 50 minutes including the application of local anesthesia.

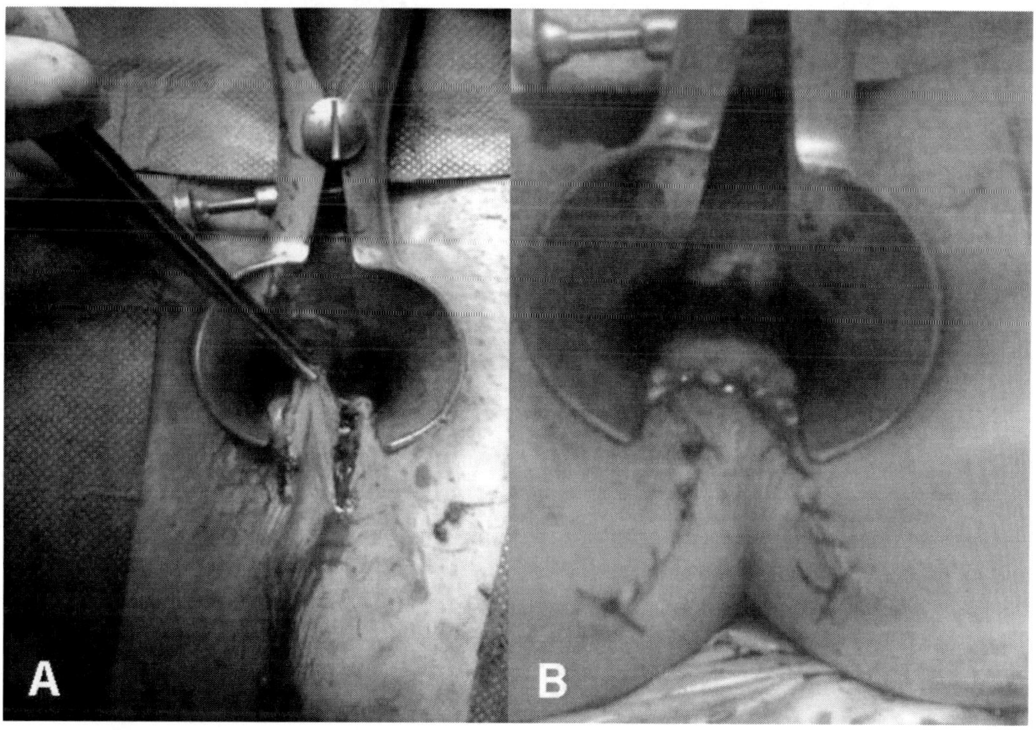

Figure 1. A. Raised cutaneous advancement flap. B. Cutaneous advancement lap sutured to the site of previous fissure.

Postoperative Course and Assessment

Postoperative wound care included warm sitz bath twice daily and following each bowel movement. All patients were discharged on the 1st POD. During in-hospital stay pain management involved iv administration of lornoxicam (Xefo, Nycomed Hellas Inc, Athens, Greece) or parecoxib (Dynastat, Pfizer Hellas Inc, Athens, Greece) twice daily. Parenteral administration of pethidine HCl or per os codeine tabs (Lonalgal, Boehringer Ingelheim Inc, Athenhs, Greece), were amongst standars postoperative orders, if patients needed them. After discharge, routine pain management with oral paracetamol (Depon, Bristol-Myers Squibb Inc, Athens, Greece) or paracetamol with caffeine (Panadol Extra, GlaxoSmithKline Inc, Athens, Greece) was instituted. No opioid-containing drugs were prescribed at home. Metronidazole (Flagyl, Sanofi-Aventis Inc, Athens, Greece) at a dose of 500 mg three times a day by mouth was continued up to the 5th POD. Regular diet was initiated from the 1st POD and was supported by a dietary fiber supplement (Bennefibra, Novartis) at patients with preoperative constipation for the first two weeks after the operation. All patients, though, were advised to receive liquid paraffin (Nujol, Shering Plough Inc, Athens, Greece) at home once or twice daily. Bulk laxatives were not offered on a routine basis, while enemas, suppositories and all rectal manipulations were strictly avoided. No patients required any further treatment with other stool softeners for normalization of bowel habit and defecation was uneventfully achieved at all patients by the latest the 3rd POD.

Postoperative pain intensity was scored with a visual analogical scale (VAS) from 0 to 10, where 0 corresponded to no pain and 10 to the worse pain conceivable [42]. A complete healing was defined as a complete epithelialization of the advancement skin flap. Anal incontinence was assessed preoperatively and at each of the assessment time-points using the Pescatori grading system: A, incontinence for flatus and mucus; B, liquid stool; C, solid stool; and 1 for occasional, 2 for weekly and 3 for daily [43].

RESULTS

Baseline Characteristics of Patients

The patients included were 32 men and 13 women [mean age (SD), 40 + 12.5 years; range, 23–67]. Bowel habits were normal in 21 patients and constipation was detected in 24 subjects in accordance with up-dated Rome diagnostic criteria [44]. Preoperatively, no patients reported anal incontinence. Seven women were nullipare, whereas 4 had given birth vaginally, one time or more, and in all cases an episiotomy was performed and two had caesarean delivery. Five patients had had prior anorectal procedures (hemorrhoidectomies) in the past.

Fissure Characteristics

The median duration of symptoms was 3 months (range, 2-8). A proportion of patients had failed a therapeutic course with topical cream 0.4% GTN (Rectogesic, Strakan Ltd., UK), either due unsuccessful healing after an 8-week course of application (13 patients) or due to abandonment of treatment due to the high frequency of headaches and resulted patients' non-compliance (12 patients). Forty-three patients had a posterior anal fissure and 2 had a posterior and an anterior fissure. Before surgery all patients had complained of anal pain particularly during and after an act of defecation. The clinical characteristics of patients are reported in Table 1.

Healing of Fissures and Relief of Symptoms

Results of the operation are summarized in Table 2. All except one patient healed completely within 30 days from operation. The intensity of pain post-defecation was reduced significantly compared to the preoperative values even from the first defecation ($p<0.0001$) (Figure 2). None of the patients complained of pain at the end of the 1st postoperative week (1st appointment). Analgesics were not required beyond the 3rd POD.

Table 2. Results of the combined procedure [VAS: Visual Analogue Score, NSAIDs: Non-steroidal anti-inflammatory drugs, LIS: "Tailored" Lateral Internal Sphincterotomy]

Results	LIS + Flap
N	45
Operative procedure duration (range)	30-50 min
Postoperative pain relief (pain-free after number of postoperative days)	2.08 ± 1.44
VAS score 1st day (median) VAS score 1st defecation (median) VAS score 1st week (median)	2 (1-5) 3 (1-5) 0 (0-3)
Use of NSAIDs > 3 days, n (%)	0 (0)
Overall postoperative opioid-containing agents use, n (%)	0 (0)
Minor bleeding, n (%) Partial flap breakdown, n (%)	8 (17.7) 1 (2.2)
Soiling, minor flatus incontinence (1 month)	1 (6.6)
Objective healing rate (% of patients)	80% at 15 days 97.7% at 30 days 100% at 3 months

Complications and Follow-up

Episodes of minor bleeding occurred in 8 patients in during the period of the first 2 weeks. There were no cases of urinary retention, anal stenosis or keyhole deformity. No necrosis of the transposed flap was observed. The only remarkable complication recorded postoperatively was a partial break down occurred in one case, which was managed conservatively, by observation only. Complete healing was achieved on this patient by the 3rd month. At the end of the 1st month, 1 patient still complained of soiling and minor flatus incontinence (Pescatori grading: A3), which subsided by the 3rd month after surgery. At the 6 months follow-up appointment, no recurrences were recorded and in no case was further surgery necessary. After a median follow-up of 20 months (range 8-36), when all patients were contacted by phone, no patient reported pain or clinical symptoms of anal fissure. Furthermore, no other complaints (seepage, pruritus, bleeding, or tenesmus) were noted.

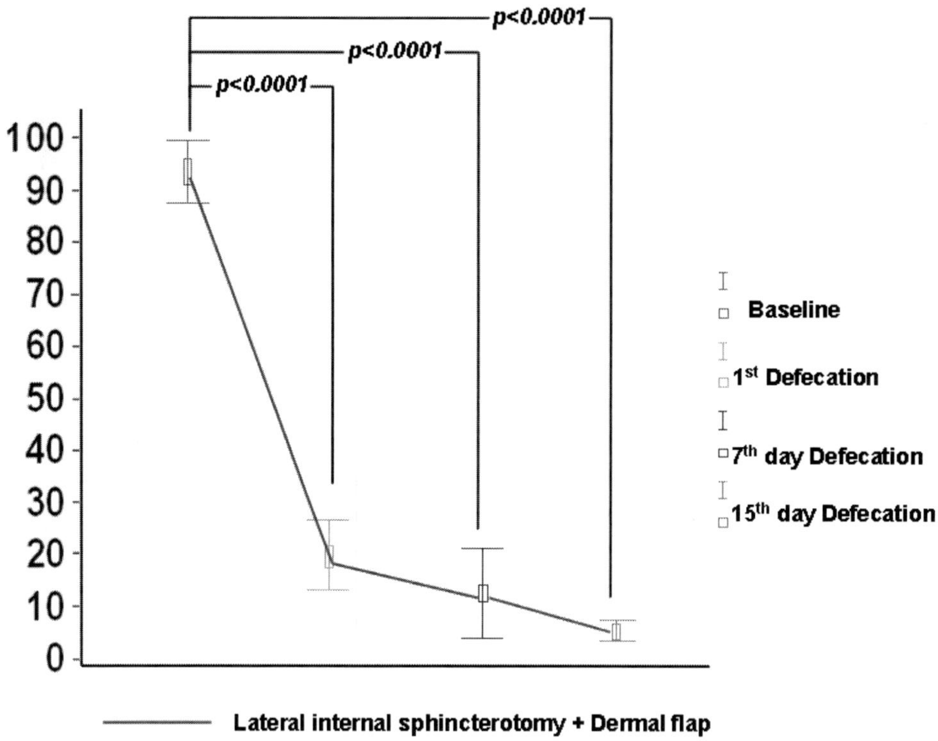

Figure 2. Significant drop of pain scores (mean values ± SD) compared to baseline values [y axis: VAS (Visual Analogue Score) values for pain at defecation].

Discussion and Review of the Literature

Introduction of anal tone reducing and anodemal blood flow increasing topical agents as additive conservative measures for anal fissure symptom alleviation and healing has led to a significant fall of surgery as an option for treatment of this tormenting anal pathology [45]. At least one third of patients fail "chemical sphincterotomy" with topical application of agents, such as glyceryl trinitrate (GTN), which is not without adverse effects, while up to half of them may experience a recurrence [1]. Despite optimal measures, a countable proportion of patients still continue to suffer symptoms. Surgical intervention provides the only potential to cure for refractory fissures that fail dietary modification and a number of topical agents. LIS is the treatment of choice of chronic anal fissures with healing rates of 85% to 96 % in most cases [6-9]. It has long been the time-honored treatment that lowers the pressure exerted by the internal anal sphincter, restores normal perfusion of the anoderm, and leads to relief of pain and healing of the fissure.

The Standards Practice Task Force by the American Society of Colon and Rectal Surgeons has stated that LIS is currently the standard of care for surgical treatment of fissures and is regarded as a safe and effective treatment, which only occasionally impairs continence [8]. LIS, though, is not without hazard. The fundamental drawback of LIS is its potential to cause gas, mucus, or, occasionally, stool incontinence in anywhere from 5 to 31 percent of patients [10-12]. Incontinence may not recover to up to 10% of patients, even after long-term follow-up [13]. On the other hand, despite the results of one study which indicated that LIS was superior to topical nitroglycerin and was not associated with any instance of long-term incontinence [46], the fact that some patients do suffer incontinence as a result of internal sphincter division cannot be disputed or ignored.

Extent of LIS, as the major cause of iatrogenic impaired continence has been one of the most confusing issues in the management of fissures. To alleviate postoperative disturbances of continence, tailoring of the height of the sphincterotomy to the length of the fissure has been initially suggested by Littlejohn and Newstead as an alternative to the dogmatic division of the IAS to the dentate line, which has long been quoted as standard practice by most practicing specialists, and regarded as the "conventional" or traditional LIS [16]. This dogma was probably based on the fact that an anal fissure may extend from the anal verge to the dentate line. The "conventional" technique used to be our standard practice up to the initiation of this prospective study in 2009.

In Littlejohn and Newstead's single-arm, retrospective analysis of 287 patients, tailoring of the height of the LIS to the length of the fissure resulted in 1.4% recurrence and 1.4% incontinence rates [16]. The authors have suggested that there is no good theoretical reason to divide the sphincter more proximally than the extent of the fissure, because if the proximal mucosa is intact, the blood supply might be presumed to be adequate. The technique of tailoring the length of sphincter division to the length of the fissure is actually a desirable refinement, but, it is indeed unknown how many surgeons actually divide the sphincter up to the dentate line. In their randomized trial, Mentes et al achieved a very high healing rate of 100% at 1 year's follow-up in the "dentate line" group, but they faced a 13.2% treatment failures in the "fissure apex" group [15]. LIS up to the dentate line provided a faster and definite healing, but it was associated with a significant alteration in anal continence in the short term. In turn, LIS up to the fissure apex was free of significant disturbance of continence, but its healing was slower and it was prone to an insignificantly higher rate of treatment failure. In another randomized study, new onset anal incontinence developed in 2.86% of the preoperatively continent patients following conservative "tailored" LIS, vs 10.86% of them after traditional LIS at the level of the dentate line (p=0.039) [16]. The times required for objective healing in both groups of patients were not statistically significant.

Preoperative manometry may be utilized as a surgical discriminant, with acceptable functional results and clinical success in selected patients treated either with limited LIS or without any sphincter division at all. However, "tailored" LIS may not always be "tailored" and may be inadvertently more extensive, precisely in those patients where limited muscle division is mostly desired [47].

The search for ''sphincter-preserving'' surgical remedies has been old. Before the widespread acceptance of LIS several historic procedures focused on obliterating all three components of the fissure: the fissure itself, the sentinel tag, and the hypertrophic papilla.

Excision of a 4-cm triangle of skin in relation to the fissure was described by Gabriel, and subsequent skin grafting of the defect was added by Hughes [17]. The primary pathogenic role of internal sphincter hypertonicity has been questioned by some investigators and it has been supported that the internal sphincter may be the "innocent bystander" in fissure disease [48]. The higher sphincter tones may be the result of direct sphincter irritation from a deep fissure eroding into the sphincter fibers. It has been proposed that the primary causative event in fissure formation is the shearing trauma, which results in a subcutaneous sinus, which fails to heal because of undrained "smouldering" infection resulting in irritation of the internal sphincter, sphincter hypertonicity as a secondary phenomenon, and characteristic anorectal pain [48].

In any aspect, fissure constitutes an "unhealing" chronically infected trauma, which may benefit from wound cleaning and/or excision. This may be achievd by fissurectomy, a technique aiming either to convert a morphologically chronic anal fissure into an acute fissure, so that healing may then proceed with other conservative measures, or to aid epithelization after the application of some type of surgery, i.e. LIS [17-20]. Even though a reliable and satisfactory method of treatment according to previous reports, the open wound left carries with it all the disadvantages of secondary wound healing. New-onset inflammation in the open area may result to anal stenosis or fissure recurrence. Fissurectomy components may vary from simple removal of the skin tag and the papilla (anal polyp) to the curettage of the base and freshening of the wound edges, which unavoidingly leads to a wider gap. The majority of the surgeons usually employ removal of the elements of chronicity (i.e. tag and papilla), which are hyperplastic mucosa and anoderm generated by the unsuccessful attempt of the fissure to be self-healed at secondary intention. In case though a more aggressive debridement of the fissure is to be undertaken an alternative other than direct suturing of the wound edges should be sought. Although wound healing per primum is possible around the anal canal (i.e. "closed" hemorrhoidectomy), fissurectomy by excision with primary closure is usually impossible since the extent of tissue removed results in undue tension on suture lines. The only other alternative surgical sphincter-preserving procedure that can accomplish primary wound healing is the introduction of healthy, well-vascularized perianal skin or even rectal mucosa into the fissure defect. Anoplasty by advancement of flaps is a technique evolved from the traditional surgical management of anal stenosis and other anal conditions [30, 49, 50].

Studies reporting use of flaps in the management of anal fissures are depicted in Table 1. Several types of cutaneous advancement flaps have been described: (i) the sliding skin graft [21], (ii) the "house" advancement flap [30, 31], (iii) the V-Y advancement anoplasty [27, 33-36, 41], (iv) the island advancement flap [26], (v) the rotational flap [28, 29], (vi) the rhomboid flap [24] and (vi) a "broad-based" advancement flap [32, 37, 40, 42], like in our series. Mucosal advancement flaps have also been reported [25, 38, 39].

Four decades ago, in their pioneering paper, Samson and Stewart established the basic principles governing the sliding skin graft technique [21]. They proposed complete excision of the fissure and the associated crypt-bearing accompanying papilla, along with a transverse incision of the mucosa to assure removal of all crypt-bearing tissue, protecting against a postoperative "wet anus". In continuity with the excised fissure and using the basic principles of plastic surgery, a flap with its base cephalad to the anal canal and a length-breadth ratio less than 3:1 (to assure against necrosis by providing adequate blood supply) was raised, mobilized with meticulous attention to hemostasis, advanced and sutured to the mucosa with interrupted absorbable sutures. Although they used nonabsorbable nylon stitches on the skin defect, the majority of the described flap techniques, thereafter, have been fully completed by the use of absorbable sutures, in order to decrease tissue reaction. The same authors defined the groups of patients that such a procedure may be contraindicated, such as patients with associated fistula and widespread undermining of the skin or friable irritated skin not suitable for grafting, female patients with anterior fissures and a small or short perineum and the patients of extremely poor operative risk [21]. According to them, but, also to several subsequent colorectal groups with experience at flaps this minimally morbid technique of fissurectomy in conjunction with a sliding-flap broad-based skin graft for defect coverage offers the advantages, of decreased postoperative pain, decreased postoperative wound care, decreased incidence of postoperative complications (i.e. recurrent anal fissure and stenosis), primary instead of secondary wound healing, more rapid healing, decreased scar and resultant deformity, and decreased postoperative inflammatory response and infection [21]. Increased operative time is not in essence a major drawback for the patient who can still undergo this operation under caudal or epidural anesthesia.

If one takes into consideration the decreased posterior anal blood supply as a perpetuating factor in the pathogenesis and persistence of an anal fissure, introduction of an alternative blood supply to the fissure that is external to the sphincter and hence not compromised by its high pressures helps in the healing of the fissure [28, 29]. Except for anal stenosis, even a keyhole deformity at the site of the fissure may be a late complication of LIS that does not routinely include wound closure [51]. Therefore, symptoms of minor incontinence after LIS may not only result from sphincter damage but also from unevenly healed anal skin with impaired anal closure. The latter may be prevented by the coverage with a cutaneous flap. Flap procedures have previously been advocated for the treatment of anal fissures in cases where incontinence is a genuine risk following LIS, such as the female patients with short anal canals and the elderly or multiparous who already have a degree of impaired anal continence, as well as the patients with a manometrically documented hypotonic sphincters or the ones with recurrent fissures with a high suspicion of decreased resting pressure due to a antecedent LIS [22, 23, 26, 34]. Nyam et al used an island advancement flap technique in 21 patients without high sphincter pressures [26]. All flaps healed primarily with preservation of sensation and perfect continence was maintained in all patients. At a median follow-up of 18 (range 2–months, no serious complications arose and all fissures healed with minimal postoperative discomfort [26].

In an effort to explore any advantages of a rhomboid advancement flap for resurfacing common anal fissures without hypotonicity in lieu of LIS, Leong et al conducted a small prospective randomized trial (20 patients in each arm), that failed to demonstrate any significant differences in outcomes relating to fissure healing, postoperative continence and patients' satisfaction [24]. Since then, the utility of flaps in the treatment of commonly encountered anal fissures was assessed in case series without comparison to other modalities [28-37, 40-42]. Giordano et al prospectively analyzed the outcomes of a simple cutaneous advancement flap anoplasty (SCAFA) on 51 consecutive patients treated over a 6.5-year period [32]. There were three (5.9%) early flap dehiscences, all of which were treated with repeat SCAFA. All fissures were healed in the short term. Three other patients subsequently developed fissures at sites remote from the original pathology. Continence was unaffected by the procedure. The technique that this group applied does not differ significantly from the one we employed in our cases. It involved the complete excision of the fissure and adjacent hemorrhoidal tissue, and the creation of a large flap. Its simplicity in comparison to V-Y and rotational flaps, the fact that it is quick and easy to perform, its durability, its low requirements for analgesics and its efficacy in the short and medium term in the aforementioned study can easily place it high in the preference of the surgeons who select the flap as the procedure of choice in the management of fissures [32]. The authors also admitted that the incidence of the three newly developed fissures reflects the fact that the technique does not address other presumed causes of fissure (i.e. defecatory habit, stool consistency, sphincter tone, etc.). The latter may be partly overcome by the addition of a limited LIS, like in our series and postoperative patients' guidance for improvement of defecation and stool. In any terms, the authors, based on the satisfactory results of the flap, concluded that SCAFA should be considered as a first-line surgical treatment of chronic anal fissure, irrespective of patient gender and anal tone [32].

In line with the previous observations, Chambers et al have shown excellent rates of healing of chronic anal fissures regardless of sphincter pressures, previous medical treatment and symptom chronicity [36]. Fifty-four consecutive patients (78% with a previous failed GTN/diltiazem thearapy) underwent a V–Y advancement flap over a 7-year period. The V–Y advancement flap was performed by making a V-shaped incision from the edges of the fissure extending about 4 cm from the anal verge and away from the midline. The V-shaped piece of skin was mobilised sufficiently to allow advancement into the anal canal to cover the fissure. Wound dehiscence occurred in three patients of which only one required a surgical intervention. At a follow-up of 6 months, all patients were universally healed. The authors stressed out the fact that if advancement flap is used at an early stage, prolonged patient discomfort, multiple hospital visits, significant costs for drugs, clinic appointments and physiology testing can be avoided. This group suggested that the V–Y advancement flap can be used successfully as a first-line treatment for chronic anal fissure with a high degree of success and no obvious drawbacks [36].

In an effort to overcome wound infections and donor site breakdowns complication island flaps, Singh et al described the use of a rotation flap as an alternative [28, 29]. It bears all the advantages of the island flap and in addition leaves a healthy intact donor site. The proposed technique used the concept of a local flap template, which involved placement of the triangulated defect/fissure within an imaginary circle of surrounding tissue. This flap had a significant rotation element in design, which not only ensured a flap adequate for resurfacing the primary defect, but also guaranteed closure of the secondary defect without compromising the flap blood supply. Twenty-one patients with chronic anal fissures, having previously failed chemical sphincterotomy were treated with rotation flap from perianal skin. Seventeen patients had complete resolution of symptoms, two patients with previous perianal surgery developed donor site complications and no patient suffered continence defects after surgery.

Patel et al carried out a retrospective analysis of the results of fissurectomy and anocutaneous advancement flap (AAF) compared to LIS [40]. Fifty patients underwent AAF and a further 50 cases were chosen who had undergone LIS over the same time period. Healing of fissure was achieved in 96% of patients after AAF and 88% after LIS (p=0.27). LIS was associated with a not significantly increased incidence of readmission with infection and pain (8% vs 4%). There was no incidence of fecal incontinence in either group. In conclusion, AAF was associated with a higher incidence of symptomatic relief and fissure healing and lower incidence of complications when compared with LIS [40].

Table 3. Cardinal results and conclusions derived from studies involving a flap for the treatment of chronic anal fissures in this review [pt(s): patient(s), LIS: Lateral Internal Sphincterotomy, GIQLI: Gastrointestinal Quality of Life Index]

Study (ref), year	Study type	Study details	Fissure healing	Recurrence	Follow-up	Complications	Remarks
Samson and Stewart (21), 1970	Single arm, prospective, non-randomised	2072 pts; sliding skin grfat	99.5%	0.5%		Minimal slough of flap (2.4%); Readmission for excision of unhealed area (10 pts); Mild anal stenosis (7 pts)	Some painful inflammation at nonabsorbable sutures closing graft defect (4th-5th POD)
Pescatori et al., (22, 23), 1991	Comparative observational study	39 pts, LIS (increased anal tone) vs 13 pts, fissurectomy with anoplasty (normal, decreased anal tone)		4 pts after LIS vs 0 pts after anoplasty		115 with worsened continence after LIS (4% with soiling) vs 0% after anoplasty	
Leong & Seow-Choen (24), 1995	Double arm, prospective, randomized	20 pts, LIS vs 20 pts, advancement rhomboid flap	85%		Median: 16 weeks (range: 6-40)		Incontinence, 0%; 2 of 3 patients with unhealed fissure after flap underwent LIS; Dissatisfied pts, 15% after LIS vs 15% after flap
Di Castro et al., (25), 1997	Single arm, prospective, non-randomised	195 pts, fissurectomy with midline sphincterotomy and anoplasty with mucosal flap (FPSA)	100% at 4 weeks			Keyhole deformity (11.3%); Serosanguineous discharge for 15 days	Incontinence, 0%
Nyam et al., (26), 1995	Single arm, prospective, non-randomised	21 pts (14 with "weak" sphincter, 7 after failed LIS); island advancement flap	100%		Median: 18 months (range: 2-28)	Contracture in donor site requiring surgical correction (1 pt); Mild discomfort at donor site (2 pts)	Incontinence, 0%
Kenefick et al., (27), 2002	Single arm, prospective, non-randomised	8 pts with recurrent fissures and decreased resting anal pressure; advancement V-Y anoplasty	87.5%		Median: 7 months (range: 2-22)		Donor site complications, 0% ; Flap dehiscence, 0% ; Unhealed fissure, 1 pt with Crohn's disease

Table 3. (Continued)

Study (ref), year	Study type	Study details	Fissure healing	Recurrence	Follow-up	Complications	Remarks
Singh et al., (28, 29), 2005	Single arm, prospective, non-randomised	21 pts; Rotational flap	81%		3 months	Flap dehiscence (2 pts)	No new-onset incontinence Overall satisfaction, 81%
Owen et al., (30), 2006	Mixed population observation study	4 pts ; House advancement flaps	100%		Median: 37 months (range:25-84)		
Alver et al., (31), 2008	Mixed population observation study	14 pts; House advancement flaps	100%		Median: 26.4 months (range: 1–46)		
Giordano et al., (32), 2009	Single arm, prospective, non-randomised	51 pts; Simple cutaneous advancement flap anoplasty (SCAFA)	98% at 2 months 100% at 4 months	0%	Median: 6 months (range: 3–27)	Urinary retention (2 pts); Postoperative bleeding (4 pts); Flap dehiscence (3 pts); Continuing anal pain (1 pt)	3/51 developed new fissures at new locations; Incontinence, 0%; 3 pts with flap dehiscence treated with repeat SCAFA
Pati et al., (33), 2010	Single arm, prospective, non-randomised	10 pts with anterior fissures and hypertonic sphincter; advancement V-Y anoplasty with fissurectomy and injection of botulinum toxin	100% at 30 days	0%	12 months	Donor site infections (2 pts); Partial break down (1 pt)	Complications treated conservatively; 1 pt with new-onset incontinence at 12 months
Pati et al., (34), 2010	Single arm, prospective, non-randomised	16 female pts without hypertonic sphincter; advancement V-Y anoplasty with fissurectomy	100% at 30 days	0%	12 months	Donor site infections (2 pts); Partial break down (1 pt)	2 pts with new-onset incontinence at 1 month; No new-onset incontinence at 6 and 12 months
Pati et al., (35), 2010	Single arm, prospective,	26 pts without hypertonic sphincter;	100% at 30 days	0%	12 months	Donor site infections (2 pts); partial break down	Complications treated conservatively; 1 pt with

Study (ref), year	Study type	Study details	Fissure healing	Recurrence	Follow-up	Complications	Remarks
	non-randomised	advancement V-Y anoplasty with fissurectomy				(1 pt)	new-onset incontinence at 12 months
Chambers et al., (36), 2010	Single arm, prospective, non-randomised	54 pts; advancement V-Y anoplasty ± fissurectomy	98.2% at 6 months		6 months	Minor bleeding (4 pts); Wound dehiscence (3 pts)	One pt with non-healing underwent repeat flap
Hancke et al., (37), 2010	Comparative prospective non-randomised	30 pts, LIS vs 30 pts, dermal flap coverage (DFC)	100%	0%	Mean ± SD: 78.5 ± 6.9 months	At long-term follow-up: Minor bleeding, itching, pain, and anal discharge (29.4%); Soiling (1 pt)	Less postoperative symptoms and less minor incontinence after DFC ($p<0.05$)
Wang et al., (38), 2011	Double arm, prospective, randomized	120 pts; fissurectomy vs mucosal advancement flap anoplasty	100% at 6 weeks, time: 17.22 ± 4.41 days	0% at 6 weeks	6 weeks	0% at 6 weeks	Time of wound healing and pain relief at anoplasty group were better than the fissurectomy group No differences at 6th week No differences in relieving anal canal pressure
Ouaïssi et al., (39), 2011	Single arm, prospective, non-randomised	26 pts; transanal mucosal advancement flap anoplasty (MAAP)	100%	0%	24 months	Perianal abscess 3 weeks after MAAP (1 pt)	Abscess treated surgically; Incontinence, 0%
Patel et al., (40), 2011	Retrospective comparative, non-randomised	50 pts, LIS vs 50 pts, anal advancement flap (AAF)	96% after AAF vs 88% after LIS ($p=0.27$)		Mean (±SD): 20±12 months in AAF group vs 22± 12.5 months in LIS group	Superficial infection (2 pts); Flap breakdown (2 pts); Pain requiring readmission (1 pt)	Incontinence, 0%; Resolution of symptoms: 90% after AAF vs 72% after LIS ($p=0.04$); More postoperative complications after LIS (18% vs 10%, $p=0.25$); More readmissions with infection and pain after LIS (8% vs 4%, $p=0.35$)

Table 3. (Continued)

Study (ref), year	Study type	Study details	Fissure healing	Recurrence	Follow-up	Complications	Remarks
Magdy et al., (41), 2012	Three arm, prospective, randomized	50 pts, conventional LIS vs 50 pts, V-Y advancement flap (flap) vs 50 pts, combined “tailored” LIS with V-Y advancement flap (LIS+flap)	84 % after LIS vs 48% after flap vs 94 % after LIS+flap (p<0.001)	4 % after LIS vs 22% after flap vs 2 % after LIS+flap (p<0.01)	12 months	Incontinence rate: 14 % after LIS vs 0 % after flap vs 2 % after LIS+flap (p=0.03); Complications: 4 % after LIS vs 10 % after flap vs 12 % after LIS+flap (p=0.22); Flap ischemia/ disruption: 0 pts after LIS vs 5 pts after flap vs 3 pts after LIS+flap	Pain relieved (days): 5.1±2.7 (3–22) after LIS vs 6.9±5.6 (3–22) after flap vs 4.2±3.42 (2–19) after LIS+flap (p= 0.0001); Patient satisfaction after 1 year: 88 % after LIS vs 70% after flap vs 96 % after LIS+flap (p= 0.016); GIQLI scores 1 year postoperatively: 120.4±4.8 after LIS vs 118.2±8 after flap vs 133.3±4.8 after LIS+flap (p=0.0001)
Abramowitz et al., (42), 2012	Prospective, observational, multicentre	264 pts, fissurectomy; 257 pts (83%) with anoplasty	100% (median: 7.5 weeks); Median time to healing: 7.5 weeks (range 2-36) with anoplasty vs 7 weeks (range 2-20) without anoplasty	0	12 months	Complications: 3% after fissurectomy with anoplasty vs 10% after fissurectomy alone (non-significant); Late complications (anoplasty): local infection requiring surgical intervention (n=1), an unspecified event (n=1); De novo anal incontinence: 7% at 1 year	Postoperative decrease of constipation score (p<0.001); Postoperative non-significant increase of Wexner incontinence score; Preoperative incontinence disappeared in 15% of pts; All SF-36 domains significantly improved; Anoplasty did not impact any result
Present series	Single arm, prospective, non-randomised	45 pts; “tailored” LIS, fissurectomy, cutaneous advancement flap	80% at 15 days; 97.7% at 30 days; 100% at 3 months	0	20 months (range 8-36)	Minor bleeding (8 pts); Partial flap breakdown (1 pt); Soiling, minor flatus incontinence, 1 month (1 pt)	

Supporting evidence in favor of the flap was derived from a non-randomised comparative study between dermal flap coverage (DFC) and LIS with a long-term follow-up available (70-94 months) [37]. Hancke et al constructed a flap similar to the one described by Giordano et al and the one applied in our combined technique [32]. Comparison of 30 LIS and 30 DFC patients revealed that, irrespective of the fissures' healing at the entire group of patients, 20% of LIS but none of the DFC patients had symptoms of mild anal incontinence ($p<0.05$). At the end of the follow-up, 47.6% of LIS and 5.8% of DFC patients had mild anal incontinence ($p<0.05$). It was apparently concluded that the DFC procedure appears to be efficacious without an increased risk of incontinence and with results comparable to LIS. In a recently published French prospective, observational, multicentre study, anoplasty was added to fissurectomy, which is common practice in France, in the majority (83%) of the 257 included cases [42]. Healing was obtained in all patients at a median period of 7.5 weeks. No recurrence had occurred by the end of the first year and, although a de novo clinically significant anal incontinence had affected 7% of the patients by that time, quality of life, as measured by the SF-36 questionnaire, had been significantly improved [42].

The excellent results of our prospective series is in keeping with the reported results from the other studies. Problems with minor incontinence episodes that persisted up to several months postoperatively, delay in patients' discomfort relief up to 2 weeks after surgery and few instances of non-healing and fissure recurrence after the formerly applied "conventional" LIS have led us to modify our technique; we decreased the length of the sphincterotomy and added an already proven beneficial cutaneous flap, which we had only previously applied in our cases with suspected or documented sphincter hypotonicity. The addition of a dermal flap after LIS resulted in excellent healing and minimal postoperative discomfort. Even though it extends the operative time, at our academic clinical practice, we have completely changed our therapeutic strategy, incorporating the flap in all cases of surgically treated fissures.

Up to recently a combined procedure, as the one applied in our practice since 2009, had not been described in the literature. A recently reported Egyptian study randomized 150 patients to conventional LIS (CLIS), V-Y advancement flap, and combined controlled "tailored" LIS (TLIS) with V-Y advancement flap [41]. Healing rate after 1 year was 84% after CLIS, 48% after flap and 94 % after TLIS with flap ($p=0.001$). The recurrence rate was 4%, 22% and 2% in the three groups, respectively ($p=0.01$). Corresponding incontinence rates were 14%, 0% and 2% ($p=0.03$). Conservatively managed in all cases, ischemia or partial flap breakdown occurred in 5 patients after flap and 3 patients after TLIS with flap. Patients' satisfaction rate after 1 year differed significantly among the three groups, with an 88% rate of satisfaction observed with the CLIS procedure, 70% with the flap and 96% in TLIS with flap. Total quality of life scores differed significantly among the three groups at 1-year follow-up ($p=0.0001$), with the highest scores in patients who received the TLIS with the flap. TLIS with the addition of a V-Y advancement flap appeared to produce the greatest healing rate, with the fewest complications and less rate of recurrence, while it was associated with the best patients' quality of life [41]. The main drawbacks for the V-Y flap alone were the high incidence of recurrence and the slower rate of healing. The authors remarked that adding tailored sphincterotomy to V-Y flap anoplasty increased the healing power up to 96 % and decreased the recurrence rate to 2 % [41]. TLIS may act by lowering the pressure exerted by the internal anal sphincter, restoring normal perfusion of the anoderm, and leading to rapid healing of the V-Y flap and fissure. These observations are in agreement with the good results succeeded with our technique, which differed, though, at the type of flap constructed.

In our study sphincter pressures were not formally assessed. In the past, during the era when conventional LIS used to be the primary treatment for fissures in our practice an anal manometry was undertaken in cases of recurrent fissures or in cases with high suspicion for sphincter decreased tone in order to avoid LIS and to use only an advancement flap. Otherwise, during the last three years, anal manometry was performed in 5 multiparrous women (not included in the current series) with clinically "weak" sphincter and preoperative episodes of minor incontinence, in order to totally eliminate even the limited "tailored" sphincterotomy. However, it has to be assumed that in our sample, there should be patients with high- and low-pressure sphincters. It is known that chronic fissures co-exist with low or low normal resting pressures in up to 19% of men and 42% of women [52]. In cases where manometry is not readily available for all patients, the limitation of the extent or, even the elimination of LIS (when predicting postoperative continence disturbances), along with a flap coverage may protect patients from adverse occurrences at their defecatory function. On the other hand, preoperative manometry, if always available, may more accurately subselect patients for the need or not of the LIS, when applying a flap procedure [22]. Otherwise, except for the special circumstances we mentioned, we recommend the combined technique to cover any scenario and achieve the best possible results.

CONCLUSION

Review of the literature and current results support that flap techniques have the advantage of primary wound healing avoiding scar formation as a risk for minor anal incontinence. The combination of LIS, fissurectomy and flap coverage may be considered pathogenesis-targeted, since it is directed against the three etiologic factors that promote the insult of anoderm by a fissure and maintain its presence despite alleviating measures, which are the anal spasm, the recalcitrant local inflammation due to the unhealed trauma and the ischemic ulcer properties of the fissure, respectively. The cutaneous advancement flap anoplasty is a simple, safe, and effective sphincter-sparing surgical option for the management, not only of the resistant and the hypotonic anus-related chronic anal fissure, but for the majority of the commonly encountered fissures that require surgical management. "Tailoring" of LIS may give better results when is combined with a flap coverage. Patient selection criteria to determine the individual, ideal extent of sphincterotomy are still remain to be more accurately defined. When this is feasible, the group of patients who will benefit from the isolated application of a flap without the need of even a limited LIS will be concealed. Given the unsatisfactory longer-term outcome of many topically-treated patients with anal fissures, the pendulum may swing back sufficiently in favor of surgery. An urging need for "sphincter-preserving" or "sphincter trauma-limiting" surgical approach will soon arise aiming in improving healing and functional results of traditional operations, such as LIS. Large scale randomized trials of sufficient power are still necessary to be conducted in order to offer adequate level of evidence for the best approach to follow.

REFERENCES

[1] Poh A, Tan KY, Seow-Choen F. Innovations in chronic anal fissure treatment: A systematic review. *World J Gastrointest Surg.* 2010 27;2:231-241.

[2] Schouten WR, Briel JW, Auwerda JJ, de Graff EJ. Ischaemic nature of anal fissure. *Br J Surg.* 1996;83:63–5.

[3] Lindsey I, Jones OM, Cunningham C, et al. Chronic anal fissure. *BJS* 2004;91:270-279.

[4] Rakinic J. Anal fissure. Benign anorectal conditions. *Clin Colon Rectal Surg.* 2007; 20:133–137

[5] Abraham A, Ayantunde, Samuel AD. Current concept in anal fissures. *World J Surg* 2006; 30:2246-2260

[6] Notaras MJ. Lateral subcutaneous sphincterotomy for anal fissure: a new technique. *Proc R Soc Med.* 1969, 62:713

[7] Notaras MJ. The treatment of anal fissure by lateral subcutaneous sphincterotomy—a technique and results. *Br J Surg.* 1971; 58:96–100.

[8] 8. Orsay C, Rakinic J, Perry WB, et al. Practice parameters for the management of anal fissures (revised). *Dis Colon Rectum.* 2004; 47:2003–2007.

[9] Nelson R. Operative procedures for fissure in ano. *Cochrane Database Syst Rev.* 2005:CD002199.

[10] Nyam DC, Pemberton JH. Long-term results of lateral internal sphincterotomy for chronic anal fissure with particular reference to incidence of fecal incontinence. *Dis Colon Rectum.* 1999;42:1306–1310.

[11] Casillas S, Hull TL, Zutshi M, et al. Incontinence after a lateral internal sphincterotomy: are we underestimating it? *Dis Colon Rectum.* 2005;48:1193–1199.

[12] Hyman N. Incontinence after lateral internal sphincterotomy: a prospective study and quality of life assessment. *Dis Colon Rectum.* 2004;47:35–38.

[13] Rotholtz NA, Bun M, Mauri MV, et al. Long-term assessment of fecal incontinence after lateral internal sphincterotomy. *Tech Coloproctol.* 2005;9:115–8.

[14] Littlejohn DR, Newstead GL. Tailored lateral sphincterotomy for anal fissure. *Dis Colon Rectum.* 1997;40:1439–1442.

[15] Menteş BB, Ege B, Leventoglu S, Oguz M, Karadag A. Extent of lateral internal sphincterotomy: up to the dentate line or up to the fissure apex? *Dis Colon Rectum.* 2005;48:365-370.

[16] Elsebae MM. A study of fecal incontinence in patients with chronic anal fissure: prospective, randomized, controlled trial of the extent of internal anal sphincter division during lateral sphincterotomy. *World J Surg.* 2007;31:2052-2057.

[17] Goligher JC, Leacock AG, Brossy JJ. The surgical anatomy of the anal canal. *Br J Surg.* 1955;43:51-61

[18] Schornagel IL, Witvliet M, Engel AF. Five-year results of fissurectomy for chronic anal fissure: low recurrence rate and minimal effect on continence. *Colorectal Dis.* 2012;14:997-1000.

[19] Engel AF, Eijsbouts QAJ, Balk AG Fissurectomy and isosorbide dinitrate for chronic fissure in ano not responding to conservative treatment. *Br J Surg.* 2002; 89:79–83

[20] Scholz Th, Hetzer FH, Dindo D et al Long-term follow-up after combined fissurectomy and Botox injection for chronic anal fissures. *Int J Colorect Dis.* 2007;22:1077–1081

[21] Samson RB, Stewart WR. Sliding skin grafts in the treatment of anal fissures. *Dis Colon Rectum.* 1970;13:372-375.

[22] Pescatori M, Ayabaca SM, Cafaro D. Tailored sphincterotomy or fissurectomy and anoplasty? *Dis Colon Rectum.* 2002 ;45:1563-1564; author reply 1564.

[23] Pescatori M, Maria G, Anastasio G. Spasm related internal spincterotomy in the treatment of anal fissure. A randomized prospective trial. *Coloproctology.* 1991;13:20 – 22.

[24] Leong AF, Seow-Choen F. Lateral sphincterotomy compared with anal advancement flap for chronic anal fissure. *Dis Colon Rectum.* 1995 ;38:69-71.

[25] Di Castro A, Biancari F, D'Andrea V, Caviglia A. Fissurectomy with posterior midline sphincterotomy and anoplasty (FPSA) in the management of chronic anal fissures. *Surg Today.* 1997;27:975-978.

[26] Nyam DC, Wilson RG, Stewart KJ, Farouk R, Bartolo DC. Island advancement flaps in the management of anal fissures. *Br J Surg.* 1995;82:326-328.

[27] Kenefick NJ, Gee AS, Durdey P. Treatment of resistant anal fissure with advancement anoplasty. *Colorectal Dis.* 2002;4:463-466.

[28] Singh M, Sharma A, Duthie G, Balasingh D, Kandasamy P. Early results of a rotation flap to treat chronic anal fissures. *Asian J Surg.* 2005;28:189-91.

[29] Singh M, Sharma A, Gardiner A, Duthie GS. Early results of a rotational flap to treat chronic anal fissures. *Int J Colorectal Dis.* 2005;20:339-342.

[30] Owen HA, Edwards DP, Khosraviani K, Phillips RK. The house advancement anoplasty for treatment of anal disorders. *J R Army Med Corps.* 2006;152:87-88.

[31] Alver O, Ersoy YE, Aydemir I, Erguney S, Teksoz S, Apaydin B, Ertem M. Use of "house" advancement flap in anorectal diseases. *World J Surg.* 2008;32:2281-2286.

[32] Giordano P, Gravante G, Grondona P, Ruggiero B, Porrett T, Lunniss PJ. Simple cutaneous advancement flap anoplasty for resistant chronic anal fissure: a prospective study. *World J Surg.* 2009;33:1058-1063.

[33] Patti R, Famà F, Tornambè A, Asaro G, Di Vita G. Fissurectomy combined with anoplasty and injection of botulinum toxin in treatment of anterior chronic anal fissure with hypertonia of internal anal sphincter: a pilot study. *Tech Coloproctol.* 2010;14:31-36.

[34] Patti R, Famà F, Barrera T, Migliore G, Di Vita G. Fissurectomy and anal advancement flap for anterior chronic anal fissure without hypertonia of the internal anal sphincter in females. *Colorectal Dis.* 2010;12:1127-30.

[35] Patti R, Famà F, Tornambè A, Restivo M, Di Vita G. Early results of fissurectomy and advancement flap for resistant chronic anal fissure without hypertonia of the internal anal sphincter. *Am Surg.* 2010;76:206-10.

[36] Chambers W, Sajal R, Dixon A. V-Y advancement flap as first-line treatment for all chronic anal fissures. *Int J Colorectal Dis.* 2010;25:645-648.

[37] Hancke E, Rikas E, Suchan K, Völke K. Dermal flap coverage for chronic anal fissure: lower incidence of anal incontinence compared to lateral internal sphincterotomy after long-term follow-up. *Dis Colon Rectum.* 2010;53:1563-1568.

[38] Wang ZY, Liu H, Sun JH, Mao XM, et al. Mucosa advancement flap anoplasty in treatment of chronic anal fissures: a prospective, multicenter, randomized controlled trial. *Zhong Xi Yi Jie He Xue Bao.* 2011;9:402-409.

[39] Ouaïssi M, Giger U, Sielezneff I, Yawovi KA, Pamela A, Pirro N, Sastre B. Mucosal advancement flap anoplasty for chronic anal fissure resistant to conservative therapy. *World J Surg.* 2011;35:900-904.

[40] Patel SD, Oxenham T, Praveen BV. Medium-term results of anal advancement flap compared with lateral sphincterotomy for the treatment of anal fissure. *Int J Colorectal Dis.* 2011;26:1211-1214.

[41] Magdy A, El Nakeeb A, Fouda el Y, Youssef M, Farid M. Comparative study of conventional lateral internal sphincterotomy, V-Y anoplasty, and tailored lateral internal sphincterotomy with V-Y anoplasty in the treatment of chronic anal fissure. *J Gastrointest Surg.* 2012;16:1955-1962.

[42] Abramowitz L, Bouchard D, Souffran M, Devulder F, Ganansia R, Castinel A, Suduca JM, Soudan D, Varastet M, Staumont G; for the GREP and the CREGG. Sphincter-sparing anal fissure surgery: A one-year prospective, observational, multicentre study of fissurectomy with anoplasty. *Colorectal Dis.* 2012 Jul 7. Epub ahead of print.

[43] Huskisson EC Measurement of pain. *J Rheumatol* 1982;9:768–769.

[44] Pescatori M, Anastasio G, Bottini C, Mentasti A New grading and scoring for anal incontinence. Evaluation of 335 patients. *Dis Colon Rectum* 1992;35:482–487.

[45] Loder PB, Kamm MA, Nicholls RJ et al ''Reversible chemical sphincterotomy'' by local application of glyceryl trinitrate. *Br J Surg* 1994;81:1386–1389.

[46] Brown CJ, Dubreuil D, Santoro L et al Lateral internal sphincterotomy is superior to topical nitroglycerin for healing chronic anal fissure and does not compromise long term fecal continence: six-year follow up of a multicenter, randomized, controlled trial. *Dis Colon Rectum* 2007;50:442–448.

[47] Sultan AH, Kamm MA, Nicholls RJ, Bartram CI. Prospective study of the extent of internal anal sphincter division during lateral sphincterotomy. *Dis Colon Rectum* 1994;37:1031–1033.

[48] Pelta AE, Davis KG, Armstrong DN. Subcutaneous fissurotomy: a novel procedure for chronic fissure in-ano. a review of 109 cases. *Dis Colon Rectum.* 2007;50:1662-1667.

[49] González AR, de Oliveira O Jr, Verzaro R, Nogueras J, Wexner SD. Anoplasty for stenosis and other anorectal defects. *Am Surg.* 1995;61:526-529.

[50] Habr-Gama A, Sobrado CW, de Araujo SE et al Surgical treatment of anal stenosis: assessment of 77 anoplasties. *Clinics* 2005;60:17–20.

[51] Yuksel O, Bostanci H, Leventog˘lu S, Sahin TT, Menteçs BB. Keyhole deformity: a case series. *J Gastrointest Surg.* 2008;12: 1110–1114.

[52] Ramalingram T, Jones O, Mortensen N, Lindsey I (2003) Clinicians are poor at assessing internal sphincter spasm in chronic anal fissure. *Colorectal Dis* 4:1, Abstract.

In: Fistuals and Fissures
Editors: Dmitri Pavlovich and Sergei Ivanovich
ISBN: 978-1-62618-068-0

Chapter 3

RECENT DEVELOPMENTS IN THE MANAGEMENT OF CONGENITAL FISTULAE

Costa Healy and Anies Mahomed
Royal Alexandra Children's Hospital, Brighton, UK

ABSTRACT

Congenital fistulae are separate and distinct from other fistulae as they result from aberrant embryological development rather than from inflammatory processes. Recent developments particularly in minimally invasive surgery have resulted in a paradigm shift in the management and outcome of the varied expression of this condition.

Abnormal connections between the trachea and oesophagus represent one of the archetypical conditions of paediatric surgery. Management of *Tracheo-oesophageal fistula* has improved from a lethal anomaly 60 years ago to the vast majority surviving today. H type fistulas represent an interesting subclass, where there is no associated oesophageal atresia, these can present later with recurrent aspirations and respiratory insults. Thoracoscopy is increasingly being used to manage these fistulae and we present current trends in the management of these cases.

Branchial fistulae have a more subtle presentation with a small opening evident most commonly in the anterior triangle of the neck. The precise site of the opening is related to the underlying embryological arch which is involved in the fistulas development. We will describe the embryology of these lesions and some recent innovations in surgical approaches to their excision.

The *vitello intestinal duct* usually closes during development, but remnants are often encountered in surgical practice. These maybe present as internal or external structures or as a patent fistula between the ileum and umbilicus. Occasionally, persistence of the vitellointestinal duct may present as an emergency with acute intestinal obstruction from volvulus or an intussusception. Laparoscopy has proven to be a useful adjunct in the elective and acute management of this condition.

Similarly, a *patent urachus* which usually manifests at birth with urine leakage from the umbilicus is amenable to a minimally invasive approach.

Anorectal malformations are another cornerstone of paediatric surgery and in the majority of these cases there is a fistulous communication between the anorectum and urinary tract. Recent developments in the management of this condition are testing conventional wisdom and approaches. We will review the current operative options available for correcting these anomalies.

The spectrum of congenital fistulae is wide ranging and varied. An appreciation of the embryological basis of these lesions both explains their occurrence and guides their optimal management. The evolution of surgical techniques offer significant advantages over conventional approaches and are worthy of discussion.

INTRODUCTION

The following chapter takes each these fistulae types in turn. The pathology is described along with presentation of the fistulae. We review any known aetiology and postulated theories. An overview of surgical management is given

TRACHEO-OESOPHAGEAL FISTULAE + OESOPHAGEAL ATRESIA

Tracheo-Oesophageal fistulae and their management are at the very core of paediatric surgery. This is an area where death was inevitable without surgical intervention a mere 70 years ago. It is one of the most dramatic success stories for paediatric surgery as now almost all survive if this is an isolated anomaly. The most common variant is a blind ending upper oesophageal pouch with a fistulous connection between the distal oesophagus and the trachea just above the level of the carina.

Tracheo-oesophageal fistulae (TOF) and associated oesophageal atresias occur in about 1 in 5000 births. This may be an isolated anomaly but in over a third of cases associated anomalies are seen.

Oesophageal atresia (OA) is usually diagnosed at or soon after birth. Babies are noticed to be bubbly and may have froth at the mouth. Suction only temporarily improves the bubbling. On attempting to pass an oro-gastric or naso-gastric tube an obstruction is encountered when the tip reaches the end of the proximal pouch approximately 10cm beyond the lips. Feeding is often accompanied by spluttering and coughing and babies are at a high risk of aspiration.

Antenatal diagnosis is rare, however if there is a pure atresia without fistula or in cases with a very small fistula. Polyhydramnios with an absent gastric bubble may be noted on ultrasound. Rarely, the blind ending upper pouch is seen during antenatal scanning.

TOF and associated OA are classified anatomically into 5 categories. The most common accounting for around 85% of cases is a blind ending upper pouch and a distal fistulous connection between the trachea and the stomach. Typically the fistula starts from the posterior trachea around the level of the carina. The next commonest accounting for almost 10% of cases is a pure atresia without fistula. The gap between the blind ending upper pouch and the typically small lower pouch is often wide and may present a challenge for surgical management. The remaining types are less frequently encountered. Tracheo- oesophageal fistula without atresia (H type fistula) may have a delayed presentation as there is a direct route to the stomach. (Figure 1) if the fistula is of small calibre, then it may not be diagnosed for several years. On the other hand, a large fistula causes frequent respiratory insults and presents earlier. Classically the connection is higher than in other types of fistula and is found in the neck. Cases of a proximal fistula with distal atresia are rare, these have the potential to be misdiagnosed as a pure atresia as the oro-gastric tube gets stuck in the upper pouch lower than the level of the fistula. Finally, double fistulae consist of a similar proximal fistula combined with a typical distal fistula. Multiple variations on these themes exist and are well described.

The diagnosis of oesophageal atresia is confirmed by CXR which shows a feeding tube arresting at the end of the upper pouch. (Figure 2) Often, the outline of the upper pouch is apparent.

Once a diagnosis of oesophageal atresia is suspected, the baby must be kept nil by mouth and the upper pouch suctioned to prevent aspiration. A Replogle double lumen tube is ideal for this purpose. The baby should be started on intravenous fluids and antibiotics in preparation for surgery.

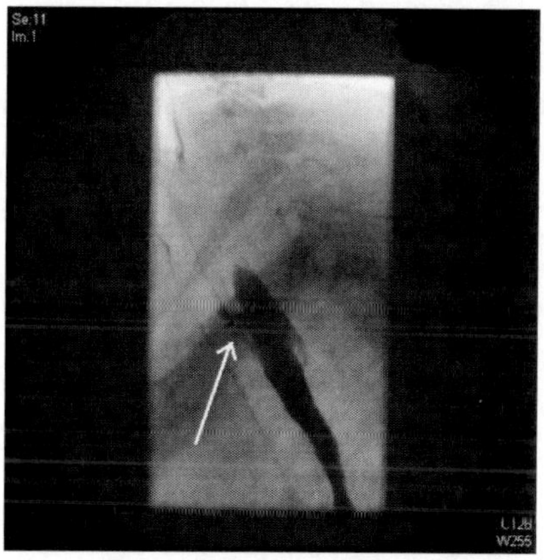

Figure 1. An H type fistula (arrowed) linking posterior oesophagus with anterior trachea.

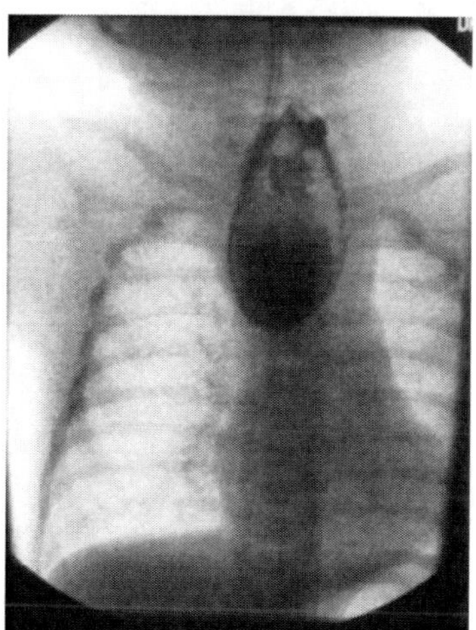

Figure 2. A contrast filled upper oesophageal pouch demonstrating a curled up suction tube.

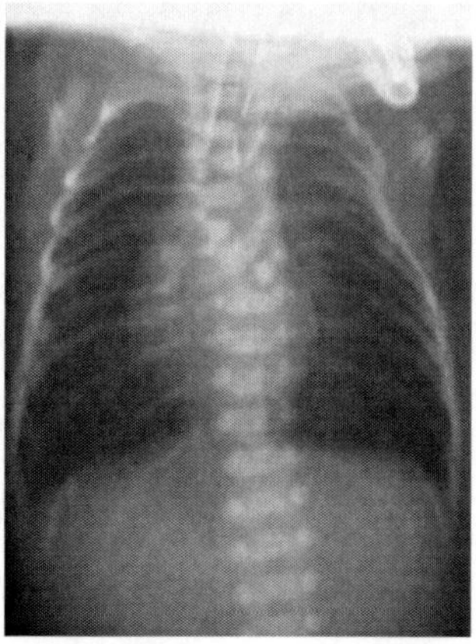

Figure 3. Oesophageal atresia with hemi-thoracic vertebrae - part of the spectrum of VACTERL association.

It is important to consider associated anomalies at this stage as they may have an impact on surgical management. Given the significant proportion of further gastrointestinal atresias that can co-exist with tracheo-oesophageal fistulae an abdominal x-ray should initially be performed. Cardiac anomalies occur in over a quarter of patients and recognition of significant anomalies has a major impact for the anaesthetic. In particular the aortic arch must be visualised on ECHO as the laterality of the arch may alter the approach to the repair of the fistula and atresia.

Other anomalies which may be associated as part of the VACTERL spectrum (Vertebral, **A**norectal, **C**ardiac, **T**racheo-o**E**sophageal, **R**enal, **L**imb) may not require full investigation at this stage. (Figure 3)

The priority of surgery is division of the fistula. This is traditionally performed via a right thoracotomy. With the baby in the left lateral position and the arm flexed at the shoulder to elevate the scapula away from the approach. The approach is ideally extra pleural and the azygous vein typically overlying the site of the fistula is divided to reveal the fistula. The fistula is then disconnected from the trachea and the tracheal end closed before attention is directed to upper pouch mobilisation. If possible a primary anastomosis is performed and a trans anastomotic tube is placed. Drainage of the extrapleural space may be undertaken as part of the operation.

There is considerable variation in the degree of tension necessary to bring the anastomosis together and in instances of extreme tension some advocate a period of paralysis plus ventilation to allow for optimal healing.

Post operative complications include leak from either the tracheal repair or more commonly the oesophageal anastomosis. These may require chest drain placement and antibiotic cover with rest from feeding.

Following uncomplicated surgery feeds can be commenced via the trans-anastomotic tube initially followed by oral feeding. An upper gastrointestinal contrast study can be performed if there is concern about the status of the anastomosis.

These children have a very high risk of gastro-oesophageal reflux, partly due to the traction on the fistula reducing the intra-abdominal oesophageal length and to some extent to the inherently anomalous oesophageal motility. Long term outcomes for these patients are generally excellent but recurrent medical problems, extending into adulthood may ensue.

Most of the areas of morbidity overlap and include dysphagia with or without bolus obstruction, gastro-oesophageal reflux disease, tracheomalacia, recurrent chest infections

The abnormal and dysmotile oesophagus does not effectively propel food boluses down to the stomach. For this reason these children need to ensure they chew their food well and wash it down with plenty of fluid. If the anastomosis becomes tighter this can worsen the problem and lead to food bolus obstruction. A physical narrowing of the anastomosis can be stretched to improve the oesophageal patency but the repaired oesophagus continues to be dysmotile.

The dysmotily of the oesophagus combined with the effects of traction on the abdominal oesophagus from any tension required for the anastomosis puts these children in a very high risk group for gastro-oesophageal reflux. The refluxed stomach contents can lead to stricturing of the oesophagus and further swallowing problems. If the reflux is extensive and ongoing then it can overflow into the respiratory tree and cause respiratory insult and repeated chest infections

The trachea and larynx are typically floppy and compressible and is consequent to the initial pathology. This presents as a harsh cough "TOF cough" recognisable to staff and parents alike. If cough is the only symptom then no intervention is required. However in some cases the collapsed airway compromises respiration and can lead to apnoeas, blue spells and life threatening events. If the tracheomalacia is at the severe end of the spectrum then surgical measures to maintain the patency of the airways are undertaken. Most commonly employed is an aortopexy where the aorta is lifted off the trachea and sutured to the sternum. Usually, the airway is assessed intraoperatively to ensure that patency has improved.

The combination of airway problems and gastro oesophageal reflux episode can damage the distal bronchial tree and predispose these children to respiratory infections.

Most of these ongoing medical issues improve with time however a small proportion will have chronic problems which prove surgically challenging.

Branchial Fistulae

Branchial fistulae are abnormal connections between the skin of the neck and endodermally derived internal structures. They have typical routes and relationships to adjacent structures due to their embryological origins. An understanding of the embryological basis of this region is essential to appreciate the anatomical relationships of branchial derived remnants.

The branchial arches appear in the fetus around 6 weeks gestation. Four cranial pairs are prominent with a further two caudally. The arches are swellings of mesoderm, the adjacent layers are made bumpy creating pouches of endoderm internally and clefts of ectoderm externally between the arches.

The branchial structures develop into anatomical structures of the head and neck. Only the first of the clefts has a clear persistence beyond embryogenesis developing into the auditory canal. The second arch grows dramatically over the 2nd 3rd and 4th clefts and fuses above them to create a common sinus (the Sinus of His) the sinus is obliterated during development. The mesodermal arches form a nerve bony structures and muscles as illustrated in the table below

Arch	Nerves	Muscles	Bones and Cartilage (C)
1st	Trigeminal	Mastication, anterior digastric, mylohyoid, tensor tympani, tensor veli palatini	Maxilla, Mandible, Incus, Malleus
2nd	Facial	Facial expression, buccinator, platysma, stapedius, stylohyoid, posterior digastric	Stapes, Styloid, lesser horn
3rd	Glossopharyngeal	Stylopharyngeus	Greater Horn (thymus, inferior parathyroid)
4th	Vagus, Superior Laryngeal	Cricothyroid, Soft palate, levator veli palatini	Thyroid C, Epiglottic C
6th	Vagus, recurrent laryngeal	Larynx	Cricoid, arytenoids, corniculate Cs

Remnants relating to the first branchial arch vary significantly in their presentation. The first arch contributes to the mandible, maxilla, internal and external ear. The external site for a fistula can lie anterior to the ear along or below the mandible. The origin is not a fixed point and can be from the naso pharynx, middle ear or external auditory canal. The tracts can pass anteriorly towards the lower face; there is a variable relation to the parotid and to the facial nerve as the tracts precede these embryologically. The tracts can emerge as fistulae along or below the mandible or anterior to the tragus sometime approaching the cheek. The tracts can alternatively pass behind the ear and arise in the post auricular area. The sheer variety of anatomical variants means that an individually tailored approach is necessary to the treatment of these lesions. The variable relationship to the parotid and facial nerve needs to be paramount in the mind of any surgeon operating on these lesions.

The second branchial arch and associated structures is the most commonly encountered branchial remnant and its typical relations are better understood. If a fistula is present it arises from the palatine tonsil internally, it passes between the internal and external carotid arteries goes above the Glossopharyngeal (3rd arch) and hypoglossal nerves, along the carotid sheath and then runs beneath the platysma muscle to emerge anterior to the sternocleidomastoid at the junction of its middle and lower 3rd. (figure 4) The relationship to the carotid arteries is fixed and due to their origins, the common and internal carotid arise from the 3rd arch so the 2nd branchial remnants all lie external to these. The external carotid arises from surrounding mesenchyme and is always external to branchial remnants. By contrast the fistulae from the 3rd and 4th arches would not pass between these vessels.

The third branchial apparatus rarely presents but again has typical relations. If a full fistula is present the external opening may be similar to that of the second type but it may also emerge posterior to the sternocleidomastoid. By contrast to the second fistula it passes posterior to the internal or common carotid artery. Subsequently the tract is found anterior to the vagus above the hypoglossal but below the Glossopharyngeal (the 3rd cleft + pouch lie below the 3rd arch). The tract then goes through the thyrohyoid membrane to reach the piriform sinus.

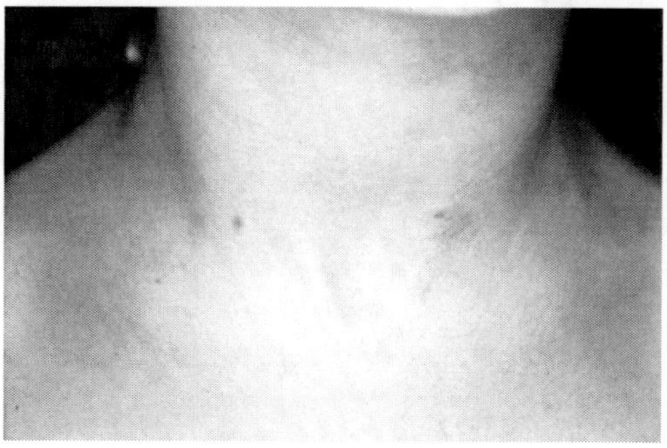

Figure 4. Bilateral second branchial arch fistulae opening on the anterior border of the junction of the middle and lower third of the sternocleidomastoid muscles.

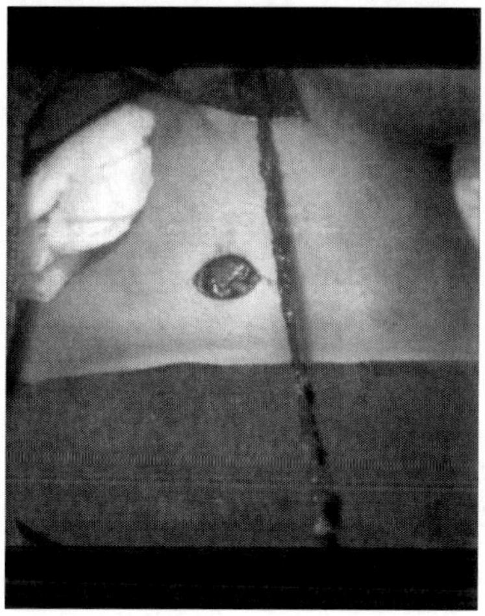

Figure 5. Comprehensive excision of a second branchial arch fistula via stepladder incision.

The fourth arch remnants are also rare. No complete fistula has been reported. The course would have to go beneath the vascular structures of the 4th arch namely the aorta or the subclavian artery. This leads to our understanding that tracts passing inferiorly from the lower neck are probably 4th branchial remnants. Likewise tracts arising in the apex of the piriform sinus passing below the superior laryngeal nerve and above the recurrent laryngeal nerve are the internal remnants of this branchial structure.

Treatment of these lesions varies depending on the anatomy encountered. A second branchial fistula may present as a small discharging hole in the anterior neck. Fully determining the extent of fistulous tract preoperatively is challenging because an empty tract is not easy to detect with ultrasound. Injection of contrast into the punctum has been used on occasion but is difficult to perform in young children and challenging to interpret. For this reason it is the operative technique that is key. The punctum is excised at the centre of an ellipse which can be closed in line with the neck creases. The tract is dissected out along its length; sometimes this requires placing a probe or stiff suture along the tract to aid dissection. As the tract courses superiorly it may require step ladder incisions higher up the neck to complete its excision. (Figure 5) Knowledge of the anatomical relationships of the tract allows for a safe dissection.

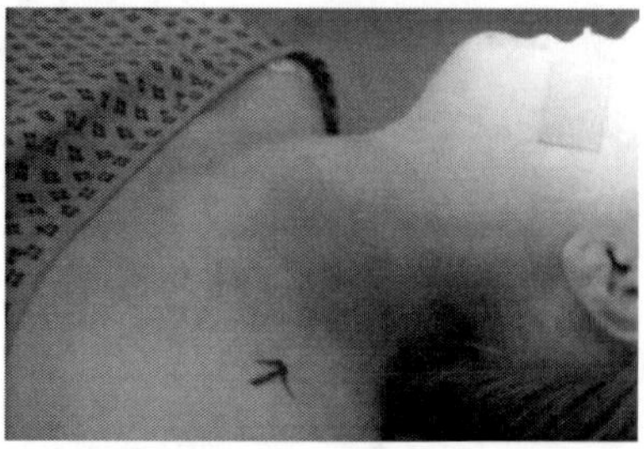

Figure 6. An infected cervical branchial cyst.

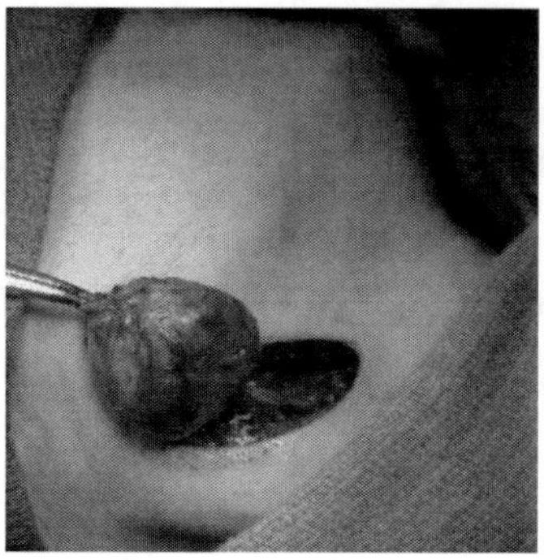

Figure 7. A branchial cyst excised in its entirety.

In cases of branchial cysts, their relationship to surrounding structures follows the same pattern. Bailey described 4 types of branchial cysts which have anatomical relations to the region of the tract encountered. As all of these cysts can enlarge with time and have to potential to become infected (Figure 6) surgical excision is advised. (Figure 7)

Following complete excision of tracts or remnants, no further problems should be encountered. However incomplete excision leads to recurrence and sometimes to troublesome repeated infections. Therefore complete excision should be attempted.

Patent Vitello Intestinal Duct and Patent Urachus

A patent vitello intestinal (VI) duct is a persistence of the embryological duct linking the small bowel and the umbilicus. It is more common for the connection to be incomplete. A patent urachus is the persistence of the equivalent structure which joins the umbilicus to the bladder during fetal development.

Vitello-Intestinal Duct

Embryology

The vitello-intestinal duct is a connection between the midgut and the yolk sac. The primitive gut tube develops in the 4th week of gestation, the embryonic disk folds inwards laterally and cephalocaudally thereby invaginating the endoderm internally. The endodermally lined gut tube is in continuity with the yolk sac via the vitello intestinal duct. The duct is identifiable as a ventral protrusion from the midgut at the centre of its axis along which the superior mesenteric artery (SMA) runs. This axis is also the rotational axis of the mid gut prior to its return to the abdomen.

The yolk sac is a membranous sac attached to the embryo, providing early nourishment for the embryo and this role continues whilst the duct is patent. It functions as the developmental circulatory system of the human embryo, before internal circulation begins. By the end of the fourth week of gestation the yolk sac resembles a pear arising from the umbilical region. The stalk connecting it to the gut tube is the vitello-intestinal duct.

During the 7th week of gestation the VI duct regresses and is not seen beyond this stage. In a small proportion of individuals the duct does not fully disappear and remnants can be found later in life. The most well recognised is the Meckel's Diverticulum (MD). This is a ventral outpouching of the gut tube which is found in the distal ileum (approximately 2 feet from the ileocaecal valve in an adult). This represents the proximal end of the VI duct persisting. MDs are found in 2% of the population and their relative frequency is probably explained by distal to proximal regression of the duct which is not fully completed.

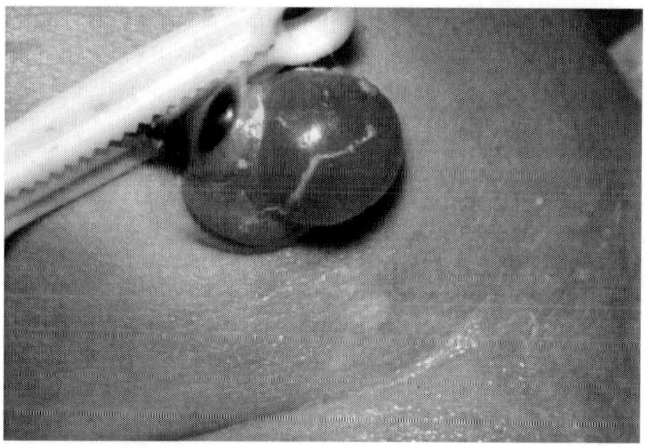

Figure 8. External cyst at the level of the umbilicus.

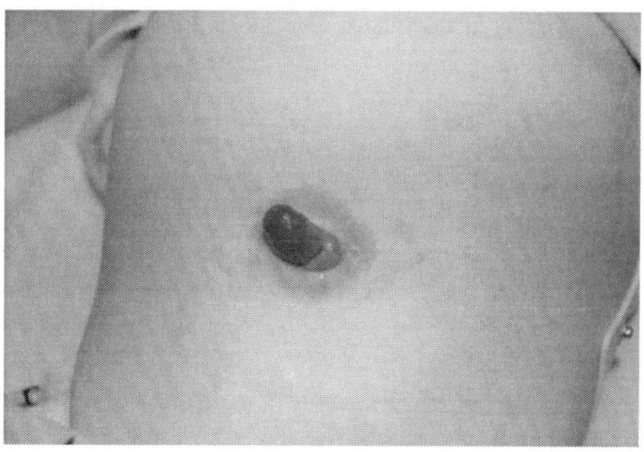

Figure 9. An umbilical polyp.

Vitello-Intestinal Remnants

Along with MD the VI duct can also persist as a band connecting the same region of ileum to the umbilicus. Combinations of MD and bands are encountered. Less commonly a section of the duct persists but is separated from the gastrointestinal tract lumen. This persistent duct creates a cystic lesion which can progressively increase in size. (Figure 8) If some VI duct tissue is persistent only at the umbilicus this can result in a polyp (Figure 9) which can produce ongoing discharge after the umbilical cord separates. Finally, if the duct persists in continuity this constitutes a patent VI duct which is a fistulous communication between the umbilicus and the ileum. (Figure 10)

Presentation

Typically these babies are well and noted to have a combination of an umbilical lesion with or without an associated umbilical discharge.

Externally differentiating between an umbilical polyp and a patent VI duct and indeed a patent urachus can be difficult. The nature of any discharge can provide clues. A patent VI duct may release flatus or bowel contents. More typically the discharge is less easily identifiable and it is the increased volume of blood/mucous which suggests the umbilical lesion is not simply a granuloma.

An umbilical polyp results from a small portion of duct lining persisting after the cord separates. These arise from the base of the umbilicus. They differ from umbilical granulomas which represent overgrowth of scar tissue at the point of separation of the umbilical cord and are easily treated with cautery or the application of silver nitrate. Polyps can be excised but when there is suggestion of an internal communication an umbilical exploration may be necessary.

If the VI duct remains patent only in the region of the umbilicus then this creates an umbilical sinus. This is a blind ending tract which produces mucoid discharge and has the potential to become infected if not draining freely. The persistent discharge is cured by a comprehensive excision of the tract. At surgery any internal communication/ fibrous band should be sought as these can coexist and may also reveal an underlying MD.

Fibrous remnants can be completely hidden and not give rise to chronic symptoms. However these intra-abdominal bands can present as causes of mechanical obstruction. Excision of the band at laparotomy is undertaken and the ileum is inspected for any associated ventral pouch. If located this must be excised at the same time.

The patent VI duct creates a fistulous connection between the umbilicus and ileum. The discharge of flatus or bowel contents per umbilicus reveals the diagnosis but when the tract is smaller this may not be obviously apparent. These ducts have the potential to cause obstruction similarly to the bands described. In addition there may be ectopic gastric and pancreatic mucosa identified as in MDs which can lead to profuse GI bleed. For these reasons and to address the persistent discharge, early resection is advised.

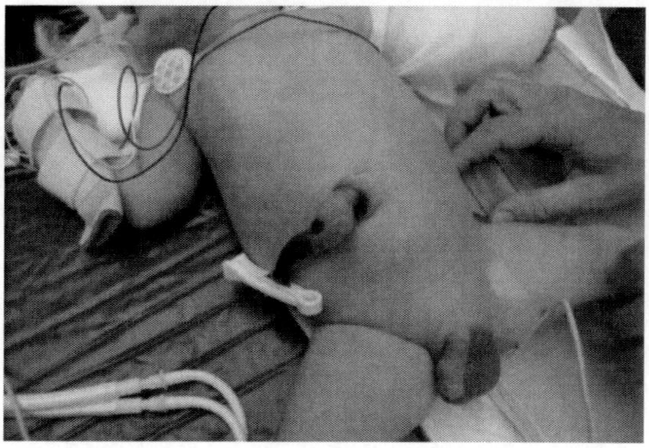

Figure 10. A patent vitello-intestinal duct with mucosa evident on the umbilical stalk. This patient presented with meconium discharge from the tract.

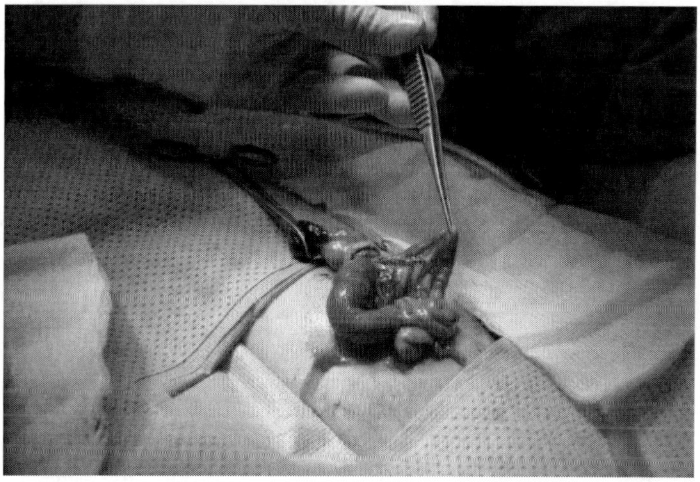

Figure 11. Resected tract in continuity with the ileum. Note a definite calibre change in the small bowel distal to the fistula.

TREATMENT

The surgical approaches to VI ducts and similar lesions need to be adequate to enable inspection of the internal communication of the tract. This can be achieved by a supraumbilical incision which can be disguised within the folds of the umbilicus. To improve visualisation and access at a deeper level the linea alba can be divided either vertically or transversely and retracted.

The entirety of the tract must be excised to avoid residual ectopic tissue and this may involve having to resect a wedge or segment of the ileum with primary reconstitution. (Figure 11) Following surgery there are no long term complications aside from the adhesion risk of any abdominal procedure.

Patent Urachus

The urachus is the remnant of the fetal communication between the bladder and umbilical cord. Unlike the VI duct the allantois does not fully disappear but is manifested by a fibrous urachus. The urachus arises from the apex of the body of the developing bladder and is recognisable as the median umbilical ligament and extends to the umbilicus.

As with the VI duct there are a variety of remnants which can persist. If there is a full connection then a patent urachal fistula is present. A urachal sinus extends from the umbilicus to a variable degree but does not reach the bladder. A urachal cyst does not communicate with either the bladder or the umbilicus. A urethral diverticulum is an outpouching from the bladder not communicating externally.

All of these lesions are treated by surgical excision. In the case of a patent urachus it is important to excise the entire tract down to the dome of the bladder as any residual tissue can act as a diverticulum which may not function at one with the bladder potentially causing infections and difficulties with continence.

Anorectal Malformations

Anorectal malformations (ARM) represent one of the most challenging areas of paediatric surgery and careers and textbooks have been dedicated to their management. They are varied in their severity from minimal anatomical variations requiring simple corrective surgery to complete disruption of the anorectal anatomy.

1 in 5000 newborns has an ano-rectal malformation. The diagnosis is made in the neonatal period during a routine examination. The imperforate anus does not allow passage of meconium which should prompt a full perineal inspection. In addition the inability to pass flatus can lead to progressive abdominal distension from obstruction.

The embryology of anorectal development and how it goes awry in cases of ARM is not well understood. Theories suggesting failure of division of the hindgut from the urogenital system have been proposed over time but have not been demonstrable. The current theory is that a deficiency in the dorsal component of the cloacal membrane and dorsal cloaca translates into the recognised anorectal malformations. The extent of the defect is thought to correspond to the severity of the subsequent malformation.

Classification of ARM is a complex area and over the years a multitude of systems have been proposed. The most recent is the Krickenbeck classification (table 1) which classes the anomalies on the basis of their anatomical features.

By adopting a standardised internationally accepted classification it is hoped that presentation, treatment and outcomes of ARMs will be easier to compare which in turn will lead to improved care.

The vast majority of anorectal malformations have an associated fistula. The location of the fistula is the major factor in classifying the anorectal malformation. From a practical perspective there is a need to recognise the difference between an anomaly which can be corrected with an anoplasty within the first few days of life and those which will require a diverting colostomy initially followed by a delayed operation to create the neo anus.

Table 1. Krickenbeck Classification

Major clinical groups	Rare/regional variants
Perineal (cutaneous) fistula	Pouch colon
Rectourethral fistula	Rectal atresia/stenosis
• Prostatic	Rectovaginal fistula
• Bulbar	H fistula
Rectovesical fistula	Others
Vestibular fistula	
Cloaca	
No fistula	
Anal stenosis	

The priority with management of these babies is therefore the differentiation between the various types. Once an anorectal malformation has been recognised the infant should be transferred to a paediatric surgical centre for assessment and management. If the infant is otherwise well this does not constitute an absolute emergency but should also not be unduly delayed as the gut is effectively blind ending with the risk of progressive dilation of the bowel. This dilation may lead to abdominal distension causing respiratory compromise and if accompanied by a competent ileo-caecal valve can progress to colonic perforation.

Before a definitive plan and diagnosis is reached all of these infants should be kept nil by mouth on intravenous (IV) fluids. This hopefully reduces abdominal distension and ensures the baby has an empty stomach should emergency surgery be needed. In addition IV antibiotics should be commenced to protect from urinary tract infections precipitated by a fistulous communication.

Once the transfer has occurred there are 2 questions to be answered, firstly if and when does it need an operation and secondly which operation is appropriate? If there is evidence of a low malformation where the bowel almost reaches the skin level, then the approach is typically to perform a primary anoplasty to create an adequate calibre neoanus. Where there is no such evidence of a low malformation or the level is in doubt then a colostomy is more appropriate. (Figure 11)

A perineal fistula has external manifestations which make it recognisable on perineal inspection alone. When these are recognised a primary anoplasty is indicated. Perineal fistulas encompass the descriptive terms anterior anus, bucket handle, covered anus and anal membrane. In boys there may be a long fistulous tract running under a thin membrane. The end of the tract may demonstrate meconium confirming that the tract is indeed the fistula. These are not always overt initially and may become more apparent over time (24h).

Perineal inspection can reveal the most common anorectal anomaly in girls, a vestibular fistula. The site of the fistula is visible within the vestibule separate from the anterior lying urethra and vagina. As the fistula is immediately apparent and can be used to guide the dissection. There are advocates of primary repair typically through a posterior sagittal approach. Results can be excellent with good long term outcomes. However a proportion following a complicated recovery may suffer from post operative infections and have a much poorer prognosis. For this reason some would perform a diverting colostomy at the time of the repair to enable a delayed repair to be undertaken.

To fully assess for the presence or absence of a fistulous opening a delay of 24h post delivery is necessary to enable meconium to be evident in the fistula tract.

There is a further perineal finding which clearly guides initial management without demonstrating the fistula, namely when only a single perineal opening is encountered in a girl. Under these circumstances there is a need to perform a diverting colostomy primarily allowing the full nature of the internal anatomy to be investigated prior to definitive surgery. The spectrum of anomalies associated with these cloaca type lesions is vast and varied and pre-operative preparedness is key to optimising the outcome. If facilities are available to perform an endoscopic evaluation of the common channel at the time of colostomy formation, then this will aid future management.

When the fistulous opening cannot be seen on inspection then further investigations are warranted. The use of x-rays to demonstrate the distal extent of the rectum relies on the swallowed air having had enough time to be passed through the entire bowel; typically at least 24h is recommended. The baby is positioned prone with a support under the hips and a lateral film is taken to show the distal gas margin. A radio-opaque marker may be used to show the predicted anal position on the skin. If the gas in the rectum extends beyond the coccyx, then a primary anoplasty can be considered. (Figure 13) A covering colostomy can be performed if deemed necessary.

If the anomaly is not convincingly found to be low in nature then a primary colostomy should be performed. (Figure 14) The colostomy should usually be a proximal sigmoid colostomy with separation of the proximal stoma from the distal mucous fistula. This positioning of the stoma reduces the risk of prolapse as the there is little slack beyond the fixed descending colon. The separation of the two limbs eliminates the risk of overflow into the distal limb and future faecaloma formation. In addition the distal limb should be washed out comprehensively to remove retained meconium.

Following a colostomy formation the baby can be discharged home and elective reconstruction planned for the future. Prior to discharge, it should be assumed that there is a communication between the distal limb of the stoma and the urinary system and the baby should be kept on prophylactic antibiotics.

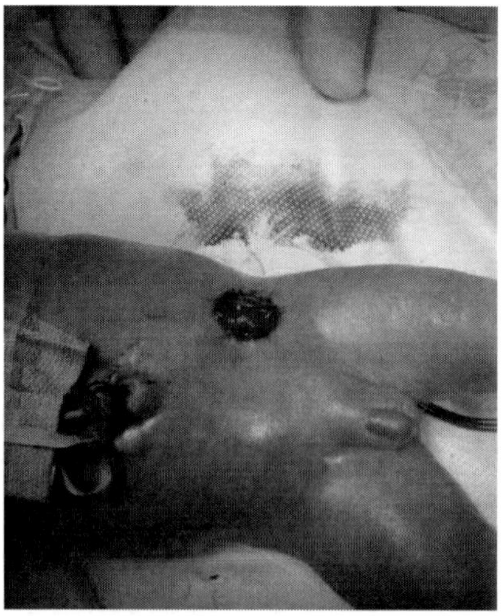

Figure 12. Defunctioning colostomy in a newborn baby.

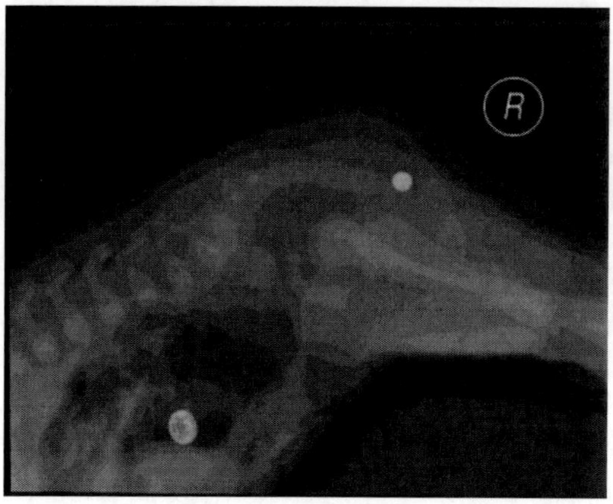

Figure 13. Invertogram with radio-opaque skin marker demonstrating low anorectal anomaly.

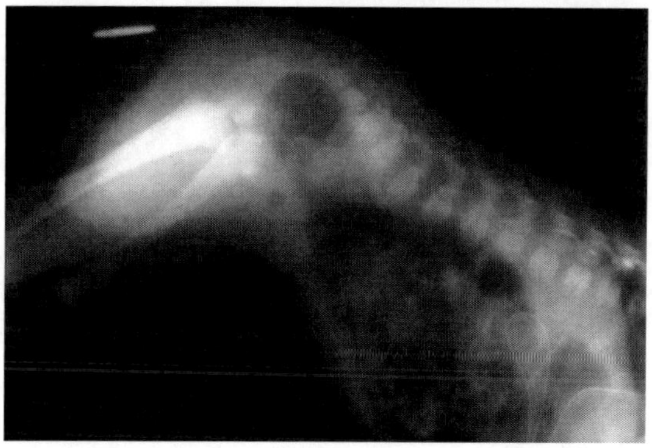

Figure 14. Invertogram demonstrating a rectovesical fistula with bubble of air in bladder evident just anterior to rectal column.

Sacral defects are commonly encountered with anorectal malformations and an assessment of the sacrum can give an indication of the functional long-term outcomes for the patient. The sacral ratio compares the vertical distance between the inferior extent of the sacro-iliac joint to the tip of the sacrum with the vertical distance from the iliac crest to the inferior sacro-iliac joint. In a typical neonate the ratio is 0.7. When the ratio is significantly less than this, the outcomes are worse.

Associated with the sacral defects is spinal cord tethering- encountered in up to 25% of cases. This can be identified by spinal cord ultrasound prior to ossification of the sacrum (before 3 months of age). The significance of spinal cord tethering is hard to fully understand. Some of these babies will go on to have progressive neurological impairment to lower limbs, bladder and bowel. However, de-tethering of the cord has not been convincingly shown to improve the outcome.

Urinary tract anomalies are also frequently encountered with ano-rectal malformations. For this reason all patients should have a renal tract ultrasound performed after 72 hours of age to ensure adequate urine production to improve the diagnostic sensitivity. A micturating cystourethrogram (MCUG) is recommended to look for vesico-ureteric reflux.

The long term outcomes in these babies are variable. Some will go on to become fully continent of faeces and urine, whereas others will be doubly incontinent. There is an array of interlinking factors which make predicting the outcome for these babies challenging. The inherent spinal cord and sacral anomalies can produce an evolving picture of neurological defects. The abnormal relationship between the bowel and the sphincteric mechanisms has an inherent tendency to impair the bowel s function. In addition surgical technique and post operative healing are likely to have a significant impact on long term function.

There are a range of long term therapies which may be required. Dietary modifications may occasionally be enough to alter difficulties with bowel habit. More typically a long term course of laxative medication will be required. There is a significant risk of chronic constipation leading to rectal dilation and worsening outcomes so lifelong monitoring is needed. Incontinence can be caused by overflow around retained hard faeces or be due to incompetence of the sphincteric muscles or a combination of the two. Managing incontinence requires a co-ordinated approach with co-operation from the child and their parents. Oral medications can be used to alter the nature of the stool so it can be easier to control. Rectal enemas can empty the colon and ensure a clean period between enemas. A surgically created conduit to the caecum can be used to administer antegrade enemas to achieve continence.

Conclusion

The complex development of humans leads to an array of fistulae arising as congenital lesions. As our understanding of these lesions has improved the minutiae of variation has become more apparent. Specialised care is necessary to ensure optimum outcomes. We have described a variety of lesions and their current management. Inevitably understanding and treatment will continue to progress.

References

Benson, Manferd T., et al. "Congenital anomalies of the branchial apparatus: embryology and pathologic anatomy." *Radiographics* 12.5 (1992): 943-960.

Garg, Mukesh Kumar. "Case report: Upper neck pouch sign in the antenatal diagnosis of esophageal atresia." *The Indian journal of radiology & imaging* 19.3 (2009): 252.

Holcomb, George W., J. Patrick Murphy, and Daniel J. Ostlie, eds. *Ashcraft's pediatric surgery*. Philadelphia: Saunders Elsevier, 2010.

Holschneider, AM; Hutson, JM. (Eds.) *Anorectal Malformations in Children, Embryology, Diagnosis, Surgical Treatment, Follow-up;* Springer, 2006.

Little, D. C., et al. "Long-term analysis of children with esophageal atresia and tracheoesophageal fistula." *Journal of pediatric surgery* 38.6 (2003): 852-856.

Schoenwolf, Gary C. *Larsen's human embryology*. Churchill Livingstone/Elsevier, 2009.

In: Fistuals and Fissures
Editors: Dmitri Pavlovich and Sergei Ivanovich

ISBN: 978-1-62618-068-0

Chapter 4

FOOT FISSURES IN PATIENTS WITH DIABETES

***Makoto Oe*[1], *Takashi Nagase*[1], *Takeo Minematsu*[1], *Yumiko Ohashi*[2], *Takahumi Kadono*[3], *Kohjiro Ueki*[4], *Takashi Kadowaki*[4] and *Hiromi Sanada*[1,*]**

[1]Departments of Gerontological Nursing/Wound Care Management, Graduate School of Medicine, The University of Tokyo, Tokyo, Japan
[2]Department of Nursing, The University of Tokyo Hospital, Tokyo, Japan
[3]Department of Dermatology, Graduate School of Medicine, University of Tokyo, Tokyo, Japan
[4]Department of Metabolic Diseases, Graduate School of Medicine, The University of Tokyo, Tokyo, Japan

ABSTRACT

Fissures in the foot, especially in the heel, are a cause of diabetic foot ulcers, and thus it is important to prevent foot fissures in patients with diabetes. It is known that autonomic neuropathy results in reduced sweat secretion leading to fissures and ulcers. Deep fissures that extend into the dermis may have a particularly higher risk of ulceration than superficial fissures because of damaged skin barrier function. However, factors related to deep fissures are unknown. Therefore, factors related to deep fissures of patients with diabetes were investigated, and the following results were obtained. The prevalence of deep foot fissures was 3.8% in patients with diabetes, with 85.7% of the fissures located in the heel. Autonomic neuropathy and angiopathy were related to deep fissures. It is noteworthy that angiopathy was a newly identified factor related to deep fissures. Next, whether angiopathy causes sweat gland atrophy of the heel skin in diabetic patients was examined. It was found that the number of sweat pores in the heel skin was significantly lower in diabetic patients with angiopathy on microscopic examination of the skin, suggesting that sweat gland atrophy may occur in the heel skin in this population. These results may indicate a loss of tissue durability at the same depth as the sweat glands. Therefore, not only use of moisturizers, but enhancement of the blood

[*] Corresponding author: Hiromi Sanada; Corresponding author's email: hsanada-tky@umin.ac.jp.

supply and external force control might be effective for preventing foot fissures in patients with diabetes.

1. Importance of Prevention of Foot Fissures in Patients with Diabetes

Diabetic foot ulcer, which is a complication of diabetes mellitus (DM), is a full thickness wound below the ankle in a diabetic patient, irrespective of duration [1]. The prevalence of foot ulcers is reported to be 4% to 10% in DM patients [2]. Once a diabetic ulcer develops, the patient's physical condition, long-term prognosis [3, 4], and quality of life are severely affected [5, 6]. Furthermore, since the number of DM patients is increasing dramatically, it is an urgent issue to establish effective preventive care for diabetic foot ulcers to reduce the associated medical costs in each country.

A fissure is defined as "any linear gap or slit in the skin surface" [7], and it is one of the causes of diabetic foot ulcer. Management of fissures has not been fully established, since there is insufficient evidence regarding their mechanism. It is generally considered that fissures can develop with dry skin from decreased perspiration associated with autonomic neuropathy [8], and foot ulcers can develop from fissures with further trauma or infection. Therefore, prevention of foot fissures is quite important, especially in patients with DM, and moisturizers can often be applied to reduce dryness before a fissure develops [9]. However, if there are independent causal factors related to fissure formation, a moisturizer alone may be insufficient to prevent foot fissures.

It is also of note that fissure depth has not been fully appreciated in previous studies [8]. We believe that an intraepidermal fissure and a "deep" fissure extending into the dermis must be distinguished, because skin barrier function is completely damaged in deep fissures that extend to the dermis. Thus, entry of microorganisms and chemical substances into the dermis can occur, which can lead to ulceration [9].

Therefore, deep fissures that extend into the dermis may have a higher risk of ulceration than superficial fissures, and specific preventive interventions might be necessary for deep fissures. However, distinctions between superficial and deep fissures have not been well described, and specific factors involved in their development are generally unclear. Investigation of the factors involved in deep foot fissure formation is essential for future preventive care for foot ulcers. Hence, the following were investigated in patients with DM: a) characteristics of foot fissures; b) factors associated with deep foot fissures; and c) sweat gland atrophy of the heel in patients with angiopathy.

2. Characteristics and Factors of Foot Fissures in Patients with Diabetes

Introduction

The prevalence, location, and morphological characteristics of deep foot fissures in patients with DM are unclear. Fissure depth has not been fully appreciated in previous studies. Fissure location might be important to consider possible factors related to deep fissures, since the foot has different thicknesses of the stratum corneum according to location. Since the thick stratum corneum has low viscoelasticity, fissures may easily form in locations with a thick stratum corneum. On the other hand, fissures in locations with a thin stratum corneum might reach the dermis easily. Furthermore, the effect of extra forces may differ according to foot location, because extra forces such as the load with walking and friction from shoes have the possibility of affecting deep fissure development.

Morphological characteristics of fissures are also important for obtaining a clue when searching for factors related to deep fissures. It is of note that morphological characteristics of ulcers were strongly related to their possible causes in our previous studies [10, 11].

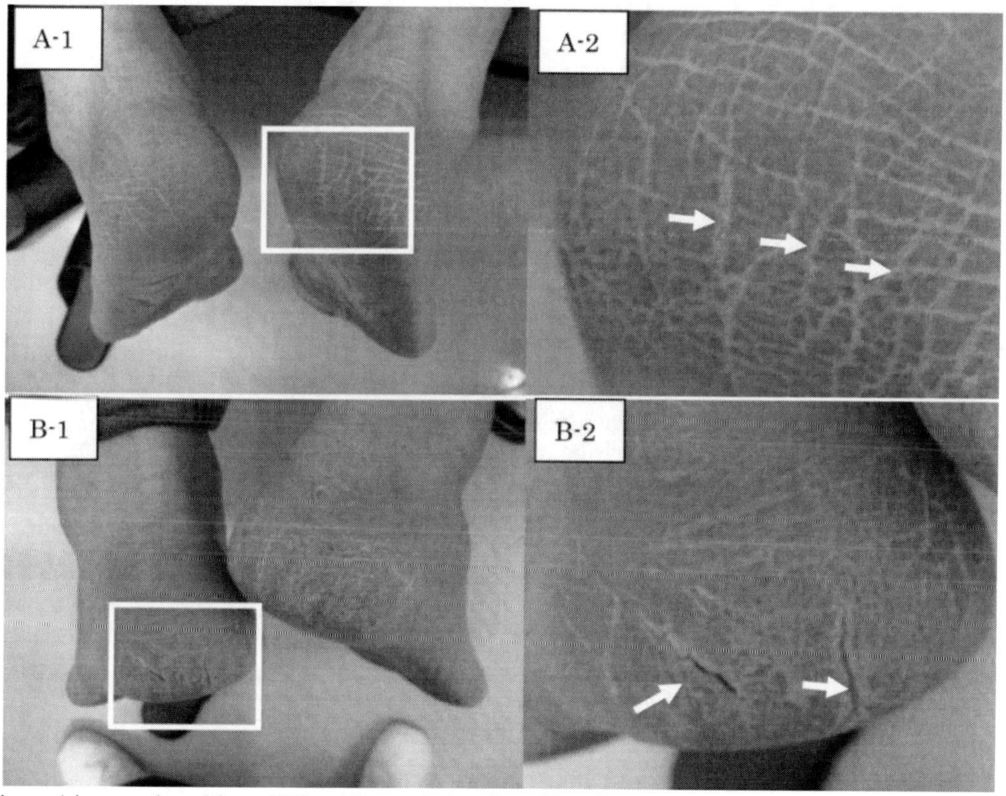

Figure 1 is reproduced from [11], with permission from Elsevier.

Figure 1. Examples of superficial and deep fissures; A-1: An example of superficial fissures; A-2: A close-up photograph of the square in A-1. The arrows show superficial fissures; B-1: An example of deep fissures; B-2: A close-up photograph of the square in B-1. The arrows show deep fissures.

Deep fissures that extend into the dermis may have a higher risk of ulceration than superficial fissures, and specific preventive interventions might be necessary for deep fissures. However, specific factors involved in their development are generally unclear.

It is possible that deep fissures and superficial fissures may be caused by different factors. Externally supplied moisture, such as sweat, mostly penetrates into the stratum corneum, while, on the other hand, the dermal layer contains dense collagen fibers and may be unaffected by stratum corneum moisture content. Consequently, deep fissures might not be simply the result of deceased perspiration associated with autonomic neuropathy.

Investigation of the factors involved in deep foot fissure formation is essential for future preventive care for foot ulcers. Therefore, the characteristics and factors associated with deep foot fissures were investigated in patient with DM. A part of this study has already been published in International Journal of Nursing Studies [12].

Methods

This research was designed as a cross-sectional observational study, and the subjects were diabetic outpatients evaluated by the Department of Diabetes and Metabolism at a university hospital in Tokyo between September 2007 and March 2008. Approximately 4000 patients with DM regularly attend this outpatient clinic. The diabetologists invited the patients to participate in this investigation. Patients interested in the investigation contacted the researcher, and a detailed explanation was given by one of the research nurses. The diagnosis of DM was based on Japan Diabetes Society criteria [13]. Patients with foot ulcers or foot defects due to amputation were excluded.

Distinction between Superficial and Deep Foot Fissures

The investigator photographed the right and left dorsal feet, sole, lateral foot, medial foot, and heel of each patient. Superficial fissures were defined as narrow skin cracks limited to the epidermis (Figure 1A), and deep fissures were defined as narrow, deep, linear skin cracks extending to the dermis. A certified wound care nurse determined whether the fissure was superficial or deep based on the photographs (Figure 1B), and duplicate assessments were performed with a two-week interval. If the assessments differed, they were reviewed again to make a final decision on the second assessment day; the concordance rate was 98.4%. Furthermore, a plastic surgeon checked the photographs and the wound care nurse's assessments, and confirmed that her judgments were correct. For fissure assessment, the investigator was blinded to data other than the photographs. Patients with both deep and superficial foot fissures were included in the deep fissure group.

Morphological Characteristics of Foot Fissures

Morphological characteristics were analyzed by "morphoqualitative analysis", which was developed by our group as a novel method of wound care nursing research [11]. In brief, the researcher sketched each photograph of superficial and deep fissures in order to observe morphological details intensively, and the information about morphological characteristics was then verbalized. The verbalized data were divided into multiple simple descriptive codes, and then categories of the morphological characteristics were generated from similar codes (Figure 2). The sketches were done by a researcher trained in this method.

Assessment of Possible Factors Related to Foot Fissures

Demographic factors, including age and sex, were obtained from medical records. Diabetes type and duration were also determined from the medical records.

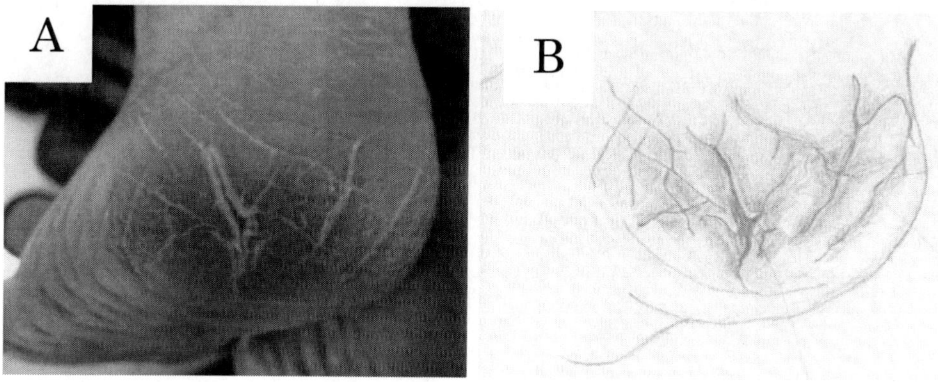

C

ID ____
The fissures are located along the wrinkles.
The fissures are long and in a vertical direction.
Brown tissue can be observed in the bed of the fissures. Bleeding is not found. The stratum corneum is white in the surface skin surrounding the fissures. The surrounding skin is dry and of a pink-white color. Especially, the winkles are white.

Figure 2. An example of a detailed description of foot fissures Verbalized detailed information of foot fissures (C) was obtained by sketching (B) the photographs (A). Sketches were done by a researcher trained in this method.

Factors evaluated for an association with fissures included hyperglycemia, neuropathy, angiopathy, and loading on the foot. The marker for hyperglycemia was HbA_1c measured on the day of the survey and obtained from the medical records. Peripheral neuropathy was evaluated using the Semmes-Weinstein monofilament test [14] and vibration sense testing; the test was abnormal when perception of vibration ceased within 10 s after a 128-Hz tuning fork was applied to the medial malleolus. The plantar aspects of the 1st toe, 1st metatarsal head, and 5th metatarsal head were tested on both feet by the Semmes-Weinstein monofilament test. The monofilament test was repeated twice at the same site, in addition to at least one ‘mock’ monofilament application. Sensation was determined to be normal at each site if the patient correctly answered two of three applications. If sensation of a 10-g monofilament or vibratory sensation was diminished, the patient was diagnosed as having sensory neuropathy.

Motor neuropathy was evaluated using the Achilles tendon reflex. If the reflex was diminished or absent bilaterally, the patients were diagnosed as having motor neuropathy. Autonomic neuropathy was evaluated by the electrocardiographic R-R interval and orthostatic hypotension [15]. To measure variations in the R-R interval on electrocardiogram, a device measuring the blood pressure pulse wave (Form PWV/ABI BP-203RPE II, Omron Colin, Tokyo, Japan) was used. The definition of an abnormal coefficient of variation of R-R intervals was based on in-hospital criteria (20-29 years, <2.46; 30-39 years, <2.13; 40-49 years, <1.66; 50-59 years, <1.41; 60-69 years, <1.25; ≥ 70 years, ≤1.14). Orthostatic hypotension was evaluated by measuring systolic blood pressure (SBP) in the upper arm after more than 20 min in a resting supine position. If the difference in upper arm SBP between supine and just after standing was greater than 30 mmHg, the patients were diagnosed as having orthostatic hypotension. Diagnosis of autonomic neuropathy was based on decreased electrocardiographic R-R interval variability or orthostatic hypotension.

Table 1. Subjects' characteristics

	n = 578
Age (years)	65.4 ± 10.8
Sex	
Male	335 (58.0)
Female	243 (42.0)
Type of diabetes	
Type 1	046 (08.0)
Type 2	517 (89.4)
Other	015 (02.6)
Duration of diabetes (years)	13.8 ± 9.3
HbA_1c (%)*	07.2 ± 1.4

n (%);
*National Glycohemoglobin Standardization Program Level.

Angiopathy was evaluated using the ankle-brachial index (ABI) and the toe-brachial index (TBI), and ABI and TBI were measured in the supine position, after more than 15 min at rest, using the same device as for the R-R interval measurement. If ABI was no more than 0.9 or TBI was less than 0.7, the patients were diagnosed as having angiopathy. Foot loading was evaluated with regard to body weight and foot deformities. For body weight, the patients were asked about their weight before examination. Foot deformities were defined as "Structural deformities in the foot such as presence of hammertoes, claw-toes, hallux valgus, prominent metatarsal heads, status after neuro-osteoarthropathy, amputation, or other foot surgery" [8]; they were evaluated from the photographs of the feet in supine and kneeling positions.

Statistical Analysis

Descriptive statistics were used to compare each type of foot fissure, and continuous data are expressed as means ± standard deviation. The prevalence of foot fissures was calculated as follows:

$$\text{Prevalence of deep (superficial) fissures (\%)} = \frac{\text{number of patients with deep (superficial) fissures}}{\text{total number of patients}} \times 100$$

Differences in the parameters between two groups (the group with superficial fissures vs. the group with deep fissures, the group with superficial fissures vs. the group without fissures, and the group with deep fissures vs. the group without fissures) were analyzed using the *t*-

test, chi-square test, or Fisher's exact test, as appropriate. Multivariate analyses of the factors associated with the presence of superficial or deep fissures were performed by logistic regression analysis, and the stepwise procedure was used for variable selection. Statistical analysis was performed using SPSS 16.0J, and the level of significance was p=0.05.

Ethical Consideration

This research was approved by the Ethics Committee at the Graduate School of Medicine and Faculty of Medicine, University of Tokyo (No. 1717). All patients gave their written, informed consent.

Results

Of the 677 patients who contacted the researcher, 579 (85.5%) consented to participate in the study; 578 were included for data analysis, since one patient who had an ulcer was excluded (Table 1).

A total of 52 (9.0%) patients had only superficial fissures, 18 (3.1%) had only deep fissures, and 4 (0.7%) had both superficial and deep fissures. The prevalence of deep fissures was 3.8%, because patients with both deep and superficial foot fissures were included in the deep fissure group.

Superficial fissures were observed in 93 different sites on the feet, and deep fissures were observed in 35 different sites on the feet. The heel was the most common site in both groups (Table 2). There was no correlation between depth and location of foot fissures.

Table 2. Locations of foot fissures

	Superficial Fissures *n* =93	Deep Fissures *n* =35	Total *N* =128	*p*
Heel	87 (93.5)	30 (85.7)	117 (91.4)	0.166
Toes	04 (04.3)	02 (05.7)	006 (04.7)	
Lateral border of the sole	00 (00.0)	02 (05.7)	002 (01.6)	
Base of the hallux	01 (01.1)	01 (02.9)	002 (01.6)	
Metatarsal head	01 (01.1)	00 (00.0)	001 (00.8)	

n (%), χ^2 test.

Four categories of the morphological characteristics of foot fissures were extracted: the mesh-shape type, the long lengthwise direction type, the short lengthwise direction type, and the crossing type (Table 3). The mesh-shape type was defined as two or more non-straight fissures; the long lengthwise direction type was defined as vertical straight fissures, extending from the plantar surface to the side aspect of the foot; the short lengthwise direction type was defined as vertical straight fissures within the side aspect of the foot; and the crossing type was defined as straight fissures in multiple directions. The short lengthwise direction type was the most common morphological category in both groups (Table 4). There was no correlation between depth and the morphological characteristics of foot fissures.

Table 3. Definitions of morphological characteristics of foot fissure

	Example of photographs	Example of sketches	Patterns	Definitions
Mesh-shape type	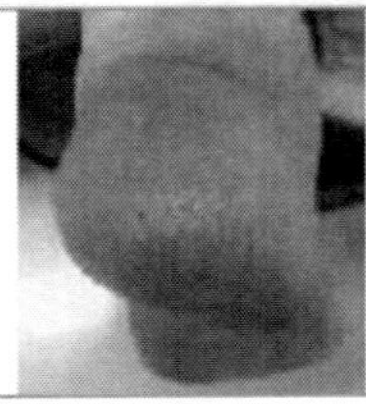		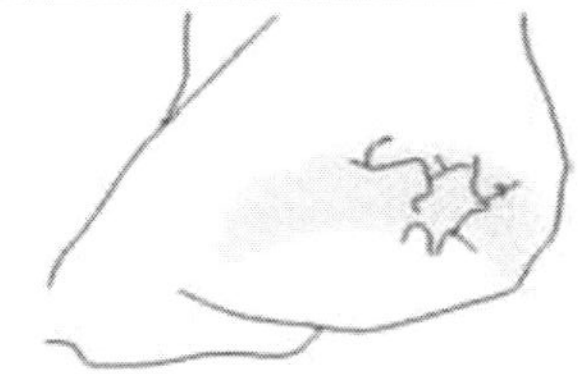	Two or more non-straight line fissures
Long lengthwise direction type	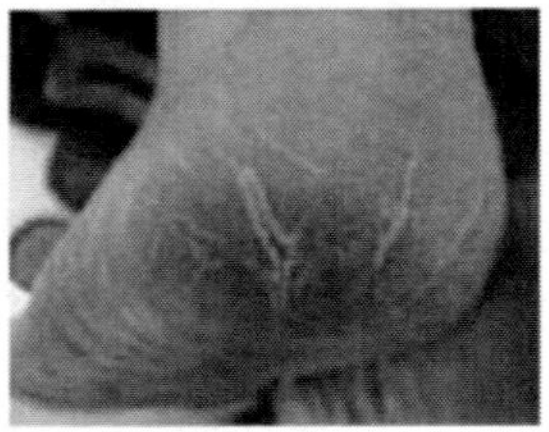	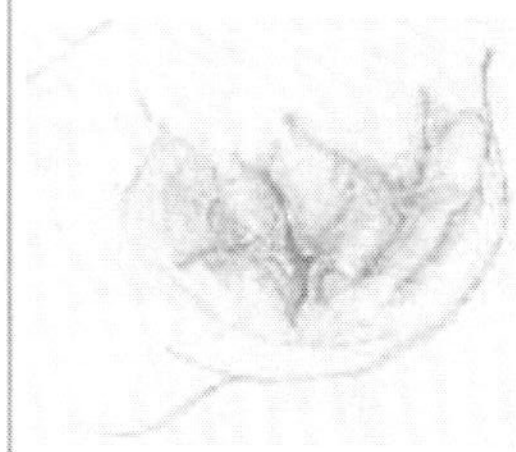	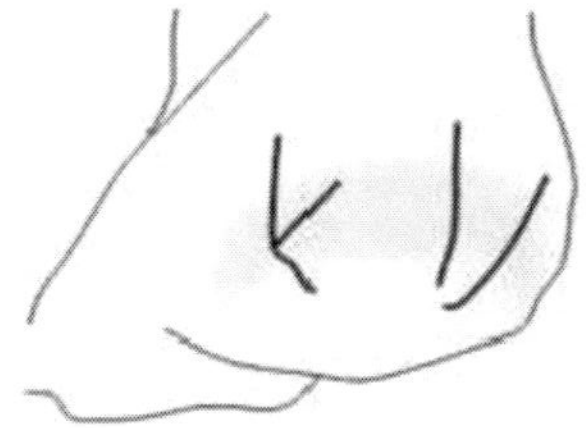	Vertical straight fissures extending from the plantar surface to the side aspect of the foot.
Short lengthwise direction type	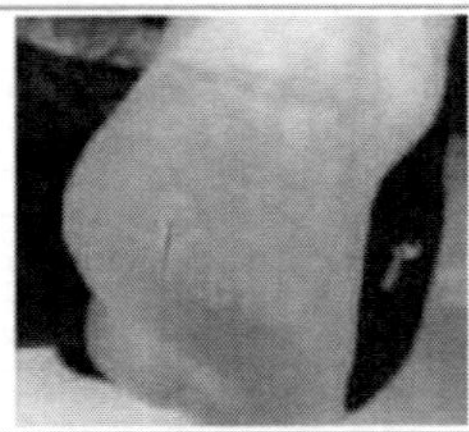	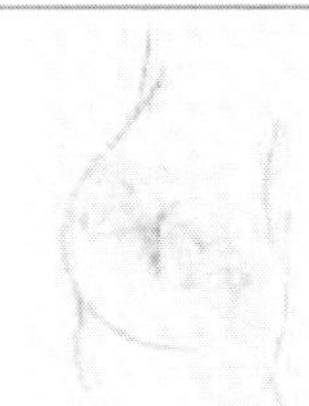	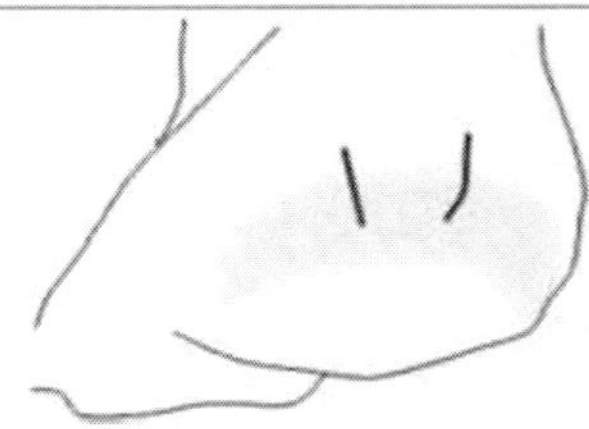	Vertical straight fissures within the side aspect of the foot
Crossing type	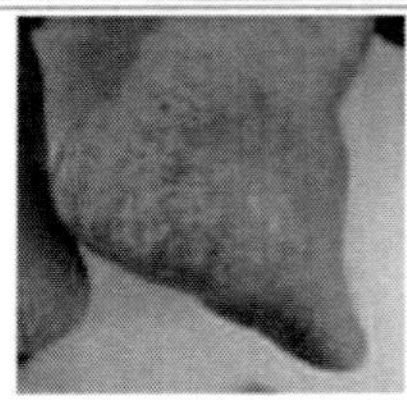	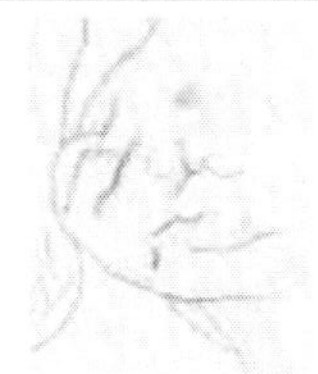	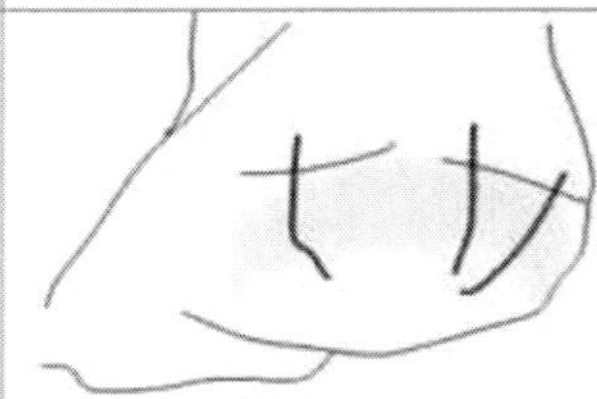	Straight fissures in multiple directions

Table 4. Morphological characteristics and depth of foot fissures

	Superficial Fissures n =93	Deep Fissures n =35	Total N =128	p
Mesh-shape type	13 (14.0)	01 (02.9)	14 (10.9)	0.305
Long lengthwise direction type	21 (22.6)	08 (22.9)	29 (22.7)	
Short lengthwise direction type	35 (37.6)	17 (48.6)	52 (40.6)	
Crossing type	24 (25.8)	09 (25.7)	33 (25.8)	

n (%), χ^2 test.

With regard to the factors related to foot fissures, various factors were compared between the group with superficial fissures and the group without fissures. Univariate analysis revealed that autonomic neuropathy was significantly more common among patients with superficial fissures (14 patients, 26.9%) than among those without fissures (77 patients, 15.3%; p=0.046). The results of logistic regression analysis showed a correlation between autonomic neuropathy and the presence of superficial fissures (OR 2.35, 95% CI 1.20 to 4.59, p=0.012).

Various factors were then compared between the group with deep fissures and the group without fissures. Univariate analysis revealed that angiopathy was significantly more common among patients with deep fissures (15 patients, 68.2%) than among those without fissures (188 patients, 37.5%; p=0.004). In addition, autonomic neuropathy was significantly more common among patients with deep fissures (8 patients, 36.4%) than among those without fissures (77 patients, 15.3%; p=0.009). Notably, the results of logistic regression analysis again showed correlations between these two factors (angiopathy and autonomic neuropathy) and the presence of deep fissures (OR 3.29, 95% CI 1.30 to 8.35, p=0.012; and OR 2.88, 95% CI 1.11 to 7.48, p=0.030, respectively).

Discussion

Overall, 3.8% of patients with diabetes had deep foot fissures with a possible high risk of developing diabetic foot ulcers. A correlation between the presence of deep fissures and angiopathy was identified, in addition to the previously known correlation between fissures and autonomic neuropathy. These findings may be important in designing preventive care for fissures, especially for high-risk deep fissures, such as enhancement of blood supply.

To date, there have been few reports regarding the prevalence of foot fissures in patients with diabetes. Mansour et al. reported a 90% prevalence of fissures in 100 Iraqi patients with diabetes [16]. Additionally, Alavi et al. reported that the prevalence of heel fissures was 50% in 247 Iranian patients with diabetes [17]. These results were much higher than the present result, which may be because the climate in Iraq and Iran is dry, and it is customary for some people to walk barefoot at home. Mansour et al. defined fissures as "any skin break that did not fit the definition of foot ulcer", and it is suggested that fissure depth was not fully appreciated in their study. On the other hand, the definition of fissures is unclear in Alavi's report. In a survey of non-ulcer lesions in 395 Swedish patients with diabetes, Borssén et al. reported a 7% prevalence of fissures [18], and they defined fissures as "lesions of the sole localized to the cuticular layer of the epidermis," which corresponds to the superficial fissures in the present study. The prevalence of superficial fissures in their study was 7%, almost the same as in the present study (9.7%). However, they did not investigate the prevalence of deep fissures. The present study is the first to report the prevalence of deep fissures in patients with diabetes; 3.8% of patients with diabetes had deep fissures with higher risks for ulceration, which highlights the need to establish preventive care focusing on deep fissures.

With regard to location, deep fissures occurred most commonly on the heel, but the heel was also the most common site of superficial fissures. Furthermore, the short lengthwise direction type was the most common type of deep fissure. It was also the most common morphological characteristic of superficial fissures. In other words, the tendency to localize on the heel and the shapes are not unique characteristics of deep fissures. These findings might suggest that the possible factors related to deep fissures are independent of location or morphological characteristics.

There was a correlation between overall fissure morbidity and autonomic neuropathy. It has been reported that decreased perspiration due to autonomic neuropathy can lead to dry skin and fissure development in patients with diabetes. Since the plantar skin does not have sebaceous glands, dryness is more likely, and decreased perspiration due to autonomic neuropathy decreases stratum corneum moisture content, which in turn can lead to fissures.

On the other hand, the present study is the first to demonstrate a correlation between deep fissures and angiopathy. In particular, angiopathy did not correlate with superficial fissure morbidity, but it was a specific factor for deep fissures. Therefore, the present study suggests that, if tissue changes due to angiopathy are reversible, not only conventional application of moisturizer, but also treatment and care focusing on angiopathy may effectively prevent deep fissures and the resultant ulceration.

There are several limitations to this study. Because evaluation of a temporal relationship with fissure formation would be difficult, the study did not include factors related to education or lifestyle habits. Excluded from this study were factors related to dermatologic diseases such as tinea infection, in which fissures may also be present, because the present study focused on the effects of fissure formation in diabetes. The subjects in this study were patients with diabetes who visited the outpatient clinic regularly. Therefore, sampling might have been biased to patients with diabetes with good blood sugar control and good compliance.

In the following section, the possible mechanism of deep fissure development from angiopathy is investigated further.

3. Sweat Gland Atrophy of the Heel in Diabetic Patients with Angiopathy

Introduction

Angiopathy has been identified as a risk factor for deep fissures, independent of autonomic neuropathy, which was previously known as a risk factor for fissures. In other words, treatment directly targeting angiopathy is also necessary to prevent fissures, in addition to the use of moisturizing agents. Since the mechanism of deep fissure formation due to angiopathy remains unclear, no definitive treatment strategy can yet be established.

Fissures are often associated with decreased perspiration, and decreased perspiration of the upper arm while in a tourniquet has been reported [19, 20]. This finding suggests a possible mechanism, in that impaired blood circulation causes decreased production of sweat from sweat glands. Furthermore, long-term impaired blood circulation might cause disuse atrophy of sweat glands. However, there have been no reports addressing which possibility is correct.

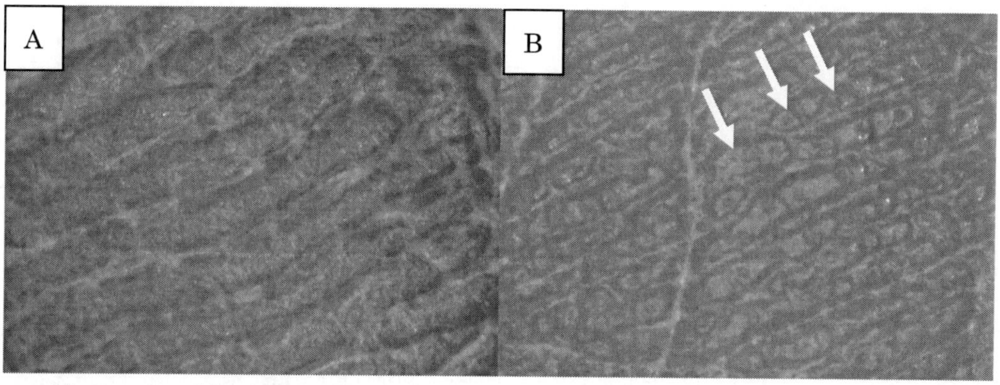

Figure 3 is reproduced from [21], with permission from John Wiley & Sons.

Figure 3. Sweat pores observed at 50 × magnification A: Representative example of heel skin in a patient with angiopathy; B: Representative example of heel skin in a patient without angiopathy; Many sweat pores (arrows) can be observed in B.

In this study, a noninvasive modality, skin microscopy, was used to evaluate sweat gland atrophy of the heel, a common location for fissures. In localized scleroderma lesions, decreased perspiration and a decrease in number of sweat pores have been observed, and they have been reported to correlate with the pathologic findings of sweat gland atrophy [21]. Thus, the number of sweat pores observed on microscopy was used as a surrogate index for sweat gland atrophy. Therefore, the purpose of the present study was to noninvasively identify sweat gland atrophy of the heel skin in DM patients with angiopathy.

Methods

This cross-sectional observational study involved DM outpatients evaluated at the diabetic foot clinic of a university hospital in Tokyo between June 2009 and September 2010. Patients with foot ulcers and/or fissures were excluded.

All information was obtained from medical records. Sweat gland atrophy was evaluated by microscopic photography of the heel (i-Scope USB, i-Scope 50XP Lens, Moritex, Tokyo, Japan), and the number of sweat pores per field was counted. A dermatologist supervised the identification of sweat pores. Microscopic examinations were performed in the supine position, with the patient's legs resting on a pillow. The heels were lifted, and the image was centered on a point where a line from the end of the Achilles tendon intersected with the edge of the heel. This study has already been accepted in the Journal of Clinical Nursing [22].

Statistical Analysis

If the ABI was ≤ 0.9, the patients were diagnosed as having angiopathy, and the data from the side with the lower ABI value were used for analysis. The number of sweat pores was compared between patients with and without angiopathy using the *t*-test. To check for confounding demographic factors, the *t*-test, Fisher's exact test, and the χ^2 test were used, as appropriate. Continuous data are expressed as means ± standard deviation. Statistical analysis was performed using SPSS 16.0J, and the level of significance was p=0.05.

Ethical Considerations

This research was approved by the Ethics Committee at the Graduate School of Medicine and Faculty of Medicine, University of Tokyo (No. 3078-(2)).

Results

Of the 115 patients, 110 were included for data analysis; one patient in whom ABI could not be measured because of pain when pressure was applied and four patients in whom sweat pore examination was difficult because of scale were excluded. Ten patients had angiopathy. There were no significant differences between the groups with and without angiopathy in the demographic factors: age, 71.5±8.9 and 67.8±8.8 years, p=0.212 (*t*-test); ratio of males, 80.0% and 55.0%, p=0.184 (Fisher's exact test); ratio with type 2 DM, 100% and 92.0%, p=0.650 (χ^2 test); duration of DM, 20.9±11.6 and 15.0±10.6 years, p=0.093 (*t*-test); HbA1c, 8.5%±2.6% and 6.9%±1.0%, p=0.085 (*t*-test); percentage of patients with sensory neuropathy, 60.0% and 27.0%, p=0.063 (Fisher's exact test); and percentage of patients with autonomic neuropathy, 20.0% and 21.0%, p=1.000 (Fisher's exact test).

At 50× magnification, the number of sweat pores per field was significantly lower in the group with angiopathy than in the group without angiopathy (14.3±8.1 vs. 21.0±16.6, p=0.042, *t*-test) (Figure 3).

Discussion

In the present study, the number of sweat pores in the heel skin was lower in DM patients with angiopathy, showing that sweat gland atrophy may occur in the heel skin in this population.

Decreased sweat function during diminished blood flow has been demonstrated experimentally in the upper arm [19, 20]. The results of the present study suggest that a similar phenomenon also occurs in the heels of DM patients. The presumed mechanism may be that, in angiopathy, an insufficient supply of oxygen and nutrients to terminal secretory cells in contact with the vascular plexus causes secretory unit atrophy and a lack of sweat production. This disuse may lead to sweat gland atrophy.

It is well known that hypoxia due to insufficient blood supply induces fibrosis in many types of tissues and organs [23, 24, 25], and hypoxic stimulation induces fibrosis in many skin diseases, such as systemic sclerosis [26]. Therefore, there is a possibility that the same phenomenon may occur in the dermis. In other words, we hypothesize that the dermis may undergo scar-like pathogenic fibrosis due to decreased blood flow, also resulting in sweat gland atrophy. These issues require further investigation.

4. Relevance to Clinical Practice

A correlation between the presence of deep fissures and angiopathy was identified in our research, in addition to the previously known correlation between fissures and autonomic neuropathy. Atherosclerosis and medial sclerosis are the most common arterial diseases in patients with diabetes. Thus, it is important that these arterial diseases are controlled by medication and/or surgical therapy. Additionally, we have developed a novel vibrator for enhancing blood flow [27, 28], and its effect was proven in an animal study [27] and in clinical cases with pressure ulcers [28]. We consider that this vibrator would be useful for preventing deep fissures.

Furthermore, the number of sweat pores in the heel skin was lower in DM patients with angiopathy. A decrease in sweat pores due to angiopathy may promote a reduction in stratum corneum moisture content and lead to fissure formation, in conjunction with decreased perspiration due to autonomic neuropathy, which has been previously shown to reduce sweating. Moisturizing care has already been prescribed for DM patients with autonomic neuropathy, and this type of care may also be indicated in patients with angiopathy.

In addition, a decrease in sweat pores is indicative of diminished capillary blood flow in sweat gland secretory units, suggesting pathogenic fibrosis of the dermis and a loss of tissue durability. Future histological studies at the dermal level may elucidate the mechanism of formation of deep fissures due to angiopathy and may help establish effective preventive care of fissures. This could contribute to prevention of diabetic foot ulcers.

Conclusion

The prevalence of deep foot fissures was 3.8% in patients with diabetes, with 85.7% of the fissures located in the heel. Autonomic neuropathy and angiopathy were related to deep fissures. It is noteworthy that angiopathy was newly identified as a factor related to deep fissures. Furthermore, it was found that the number of sweat pores in the heel skin was significantly lower in diabetic patients with angiopathy on microscopic skin examination, suggesting that sweat gland atrophy may occur in the heel skin in this population. These results may indicate a loss of tissue durability at the same depth as the sweat glands. Therefore, not only use of moisturizers but enhancement of the blood supply and external force control might be effective for prevention of deep foot fissures in patients with diabetes.

REFERENCES

[1] Reiber, G. E., Lipsky, B. A. & Gibbons, G. W. (1998). The burden of diabetic foot ulcers. *Am J Surg,* 176(2A Suppl), 5S-10S.

[2] Singh, N., Armstrong, D. G. & Lipsky, B. A. (2005). Preventing foot ulcers in patients with diabetes. *JAMA,* 293(2), 217-28.

[3] Lehto, S., Rönnemaa, T., Pyörälä, K. & Laakso, M. (1996). Risk factors predicting lower extremity amputations in patients with NIDDM. *Diabetes Care,* 19(6), 607-12.

[4] Boyko, E. J., Ahroni, J. H., Smith, D. G. & Davignon, D. (1996). Increased mortality associated with diabetic foot ulcer. *Diabet Med,* 13 (11), 967-72.

[5] Ragnarson, Tennvall, G. & Apelqvist, J. (2000). Health-related quality of life in patients with diabetes mellitus and foot ulcers. *J Diabetes Complications,* 14(5), 235-41.

[6] Nabuurs-Franssen, M. H., Huijberts, M. S., Nieuwenhuijzen Kruseman, A. C., Willems, J. & Schaper, N. C. (2005). Health-related quality of life of diabetic foot ulcer patients and their caregivers. *Diabetologia,* 48(9), 1906-10.

[7] Burns, T., Breathnach, S., Cox, N. & Griffiths, C. (2004). Rook's *Textbook of Dermatology*. Malden; Blackwell.

[8] The International Working Group on the Diabetic Foot. (2007). *The International Consensus on the Management and Prevention of* the *Diabetic Foot* [DVD], Amsterdam, the Netherlands: International Working Group on the Diabetic Foot.

[9] Pavicic, T. & Korting, H. C. (2006). Xerosis and callus formation as a key to the diabetic foot syndrome: dermatologic view of the problem and its management. *Journal of the German society of dermatology*, 4, 935-941.

[10] Sato, M., Sanada, H., Konya, C., Sugama, J. & Nakagami, G. (2006). Prognosis of stage I pressure ulcers and related factors. *Int Wound J,* 3 (4), 355-62.

[11] Nanjo, Y., Nakagami, G., Kaitani, T., Naito, A., Takehara, K., Lijuan, J., Yahagi, N. & Sanada, H. (2011). Relationship between morphological characteristics and etiology of pressure ulcers in intensive care unit patients. *J Wound Ostomy Continence Nurs*, (38)4, 404-412.

[12] Oe, M., Sanada, H., Nagase, T., Minematsu, T., Ohashi, Y., Kadono, T., Ueki, K. & Kadowaki, T. (2012). Factors associated with deep foot fissures in diabetic patients: A cross-sectional observational study. *Int J Nurs Stud,* 49(6), 739-746.

[13] The Committee of Japan Diabetes Society on the Classification and Diagnostic Criteria of Diabetes Mellitus. (1999). Report of the Committee of Japan Diabetes Society on the Classification and Diagnostic Criteria of Diabetes Mellitus. *Journal of the Japan Diabetes Society,* 42(5), 385-404 (In Japanese).

[14] Apelqvist, J., Bakker, K., van Houtum, W. H. & Schaper, N. C., International Working Group on the Diabetic Foot (IWGDF) Editorial Board. (2008). Practical guidelines on the management and prevention of the diabetic foot: Based upon the International Consensus on the Diabetic Foot (2007) Prepared by the International Working Group on the Diabetic Foot. *Diabetes/metabolism research and reviews*, 24Suppl 1, S181-187.

[15] Japan Diabetes Society. (2006). *Diabetes mellitus treatment guide 2006-2007.* Tokyo: Bunkodo Publisher (In Japanese).

[16] Mansour, A. A. & Dahyak, S. G. (2008). Are foot abnormalities more common in adults *The Permanente Journal*, 12(4), 25-30.

[17] Alavi, A., Sanjari, M., Haghdoost, A. & Sibbald, R. G. (2009). Common foot examination features of 247 Iranian patients with diabetes. *International wound journal,* 6(2), 117-122.

[18] Borssén, B., Bergenheim, T. & Lithner, F. (1990). The epidemiology of foot lesions in diabetic patients aged 15-50 years. *Diabetic medicine,* 7, 438-444.

[19] Collins, K. J., Sargent, F. & Weiner, J. S. (1959). The effect of arterial occlusion on sweat-gland responses in the human forearm. *J. Physiol,* 148, 615-24.

[20] van Heyningen, R. & Weiner, J. S. (1952). The effect of arterial occlusion on sweat composition. *J. Physiol,* 116, 404-13.

[21] Serup, J. (1984). Localized scleroderma (morphoea): studies of eccrine gland function and skin microtopography. *J. Dermatol,* 11, 269-76.

[22] Oe, M., Sanada, H., Nagase, T., Minematsu, T., Ohashi, Y., Kadono, T., Ueki, K. & Kadowaki, T. (2012). Sweat Gland Atrophy of the Heel in Diabetic Patients with Angiopathy. *Journal of Clinical Nursing,* inpress.

[23] Manotham, K., Tanaka, T., Matsumoto, M., Ohse, T., Miyata, T., Inagi, R., Kurokawa, K., Fujita, T. & Nangaku, M. (2004). Evidence of tubular hypoxia in the early phase in the remnant kidney model. *Journal of the American Society of Nephrology,* 15, 1277-1288.

[24] Higgins, D. F., Kimura, K., Bernhardt, W. M., Shrimanker, N., Akai, Y., Hohenstein, B., Saito, Y., Johnson, R. S., Kretzler, M., Cohen, C. D., Eckardt, K. U., Iwano, M. & Haase, V. H. (2007). Hypoxia promotes fibrogenesis *in vivo* via HIF-1 stimulation of epithelial-to-mesenchymal transition. *The Journal of clinical investigation,* 117, 3810-3820.

[25] Kimura, K., Iwano, M., Higgins, D. F., Yamaguchi, Y., Nakatani, K., Harada, K., Kubo, A., Akai, Y., Rankin, E. B., Neilson, E. G., Haase, V. H. & Saito, Y. (2008). Stable expression of HIF-1alpha in tubular epithelial cells promotes interstitial fibrosis. *American journal of physiology,* 295, F1023-1029.

[26] Varga, J. & Abraham, D. (2007). Systemic sclerosis: a prototypic multisystem fibrotic disorder. *The Journal of clinical investigation,* 117, 557-556.

[27] Nakagami, G., Sanada, H., Matsui, N., Kitagawa, A., Yokogawa, H., Sekiya, N., Ichioka, S., Sugama, J. & Shibata, M. (2007). Effect of vibration on skin blood flow in an *in vivo* microcirculatory model. *BioScience Trends,* 1(3), 161-166.

[28] Arashi, M., Sugama, J., Sanada, H., Konya, C., Okuwa, M., Nakagami, G., Inoue, A. & Tabata, K. (2010). Vibration therapy accelerates healing of stage I pressure ulcers in older adult patients. *Advances in skin and wound care,* 23(7), 321-317.

In: Fistuals and Fissures
Editors: Dmitri Pavlovich and Sergei Ivanovich
ISBN: 978-1-62618-068-0

Chapter 5

Pancreatic Fistulae: Clinical Features, Diagnosis and Treatment

Marcos Kutz,[1*] Juan José Vila,[2] Silvia Goñi,[1] Juan Carrascosa,[1] Marta Basterra,[2] Marta Gómez[2] and María Luz Almendral[1]

[1]Hospital of Zumárraga, Spain
[2]Complejo Hospitalario de Navarra, Spain

Abstract

A pancreatic fistula (PF) is an abnormal communication between the pancreatic duct and neighboring organs or spaces. They are classified as external or internal depending on whether they communicate with the skin or other organs.

PFs are caused mainly by acute or chronic pancreatitis, as well as by pancreatic surgery. Their clinical manifestations vary according to their location, size and affected organs, and they may include electrolyte imbalance, malnutrition, infection, abdominal pain, ascites, dyspnea and thoracic pain.

PFs are suspected by clinical features and radiological imaging, and confirmed by the finding of high levels of amylase in the extravasated fluid, which often exceed 4000 U/L. Magnetic resonance cholangiopancreatography should be the first imaging tool used in the diagnostic work-up, followed by endoscopic retrograde cholangiopancreatography, which is the most accurate method but has the drawback of its invasive nature.

The initial treatment of pancreatic fistulae is conservative, including nasojejunal feeding, broad spectrum antibiotic therapy and correction of electrolyte imbalances. This approach achieves closure rates of up to 80 percent.

When conservative therapy fails, endoscopic ERCP treatment is to be employed with the intention to drain collections if present, dilate pancreatic duct strictures and/or reduce pancreatic duct pressure through stent placement.

Surgery is the final option when other approaches prove themselves unsuccessful. Surgical techniques include pancreatic resection and jejunostomy, and achieve success rates of up to 90 percent, with mortality rates of 6 percent in some series.

[*] Corresponding author: Marcos Kutz. E-mail: mkutzleo@alumni.unav.es.

Introduction

Pancreatic fistulae appear as a complication of pancreatic disease or pancreatic trauma, either of surgical origin or from other causes. The term refers to the abnormal communication between the pancreatic duct and other organs or spaces.

The word leakage, used mainly in the surgical sphere, may be also found in the literature referring to the same complication. Some authors [1] differentiate both concepts by the duration of the complication (a fistula would be a chronified leakage), whereas others define them differently [2]: a fistula would be a communication between two epithelialized surfaces, and a leakage an abnormal escape of fluid through an orifice or opening. In any case, both terms are used interchangeably in pancreatic surgery literature, and no consensus has been reached.

Fistulae secondary to pancreatic resection (*postoperative pancreatic fistulae*) have been diagnosed using different criteria over the last years, leading to a broad range of definitions that have hindered adequate comparisons between studies.

In 2005, the International Study Group on Pancreatic Fistula (ISGPF) developed a consensus definition: output via an operatively-placed drain (or a subsequently placed percutaneous drain) of any measurable volume of drain fluid on or after postoperative day three, with an amylase content greater than three times the upper normal serum value [2].

Classification

Fistulae may be classified taking several aspects into consideration:

- Location of fluid drainage:
  - Internal fistulae: communicated with an internal organ or space.
  - External fistulae: communicated with the skin. They may in turn be divided in high (>200 ml/day) or low (<200 ml/day) output fistulae.
- Underlying process causing the complication.
- Clinical criteria, also developed by the ISGPF [2] and used mainly regarding surgical fistulae:
  - Grade A: transient and asymptomatic fistulae, evident only by high drain amylase levels.
  - Grade B: symptomatic, clinically apparent fistulae that require diagnostic evaluation and therapeutic management, including antibiotic therapy, supplemental nutrition, somatostatin analogues, and percutaneous drainage.
  - Grade C: most severe fistulae that require major management deviations, may result in sepsis, organ failure or death, and may require surgical exploration.

Incidence

Most incidence data regarding pancreatic fistula refer to fistulae arisen as surgical complications after pancreatic resection. Due to the longstanding lack of defining criteria, reported incidences range from 5 to 30 percent, figures that, remarkably, have not changed significantly over the last three decades [3].

ETIOLOGY

Fistulae are the consequence of a disrupted pancreatic duct (Figure 1). Such disruption allows the enzyme-rich pancreatic fluid to contact adjacent tissues, which become thus damaged and ruptured, permitting the fluid to further progress. Pancreatic protease plays a key role in this sequence.

Pseudocyst formation is another possible outcome of Wirsing's duct rupture, which occurs when the leaked fluid is contained by the surrounding structures. Pseudocysts may be communicated with fistulae as well.

Any pancreatic disorder or abdominal trauma that can damage the pancreatic duct may cause a pancreatic fistula. Chronic alcohol-induced pancreatitis is the most frequent cause of internal fistula [4], whereas most external fistulae are of iatrogenic origin, such as pancreatic resection or percutaneous drainage of pancreatic collections.

Other possible etiologies are acute or chronic pancreatitis of any cause, pancreatic biopsy, blunt trauma or unintended duct damage during abdominal surgery.

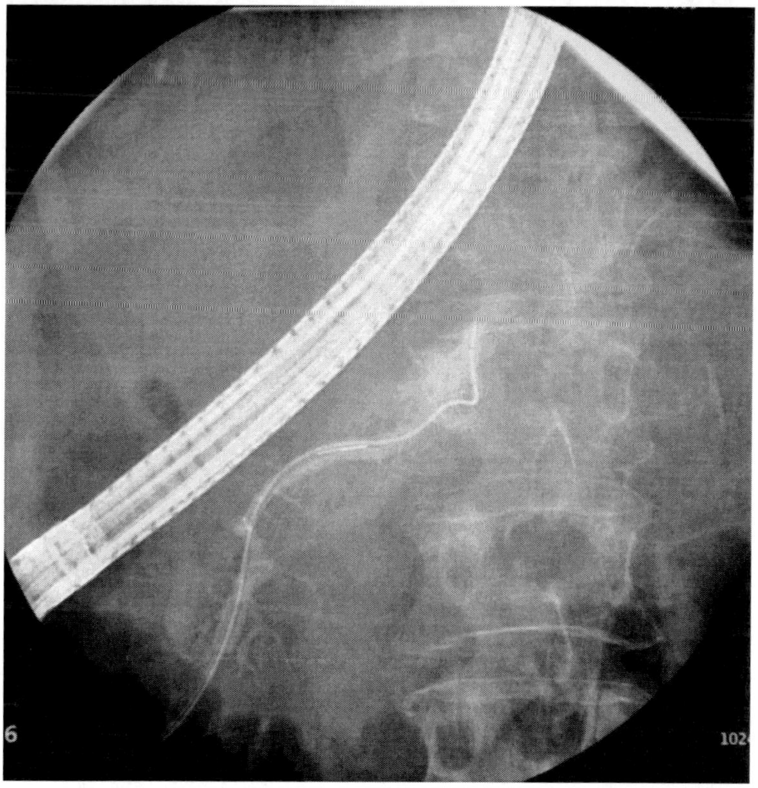

Figure 1. ERCP image showing pancreatic duct disruption. Contrast fluid may be observed flowing toward the upper vertebrae through a pancreatic fistula. The guidewire has as well progressed through the disruption into the fistula.

RISK FACTORS FOR POSTSURGICAL PANCREATIC FISTULA

Owing to the considerable incidence of pancreatic fistula following pancreatic resection, risk factors for such complication have been recurrently studied. Risk factors may be divided in several categories. The following refer to pancreaticoduodenectomy.

Patient Related Risk Factors

Age: Elderly age (over 70 years) has been associated with poor anastomotic healing and fistula. [5]

Coronary artery disease: A study demonstrated a correlation between a history of coronary artery disease and postresection fistula formation. [6] The proposed mechanism behind this finding was a hindered anastomotic healing process caused by poor blood perfusion.

Other risk factors: Male gender, [6] longer duration of jaundice (as opposed to bilirubin level) [7] and lower creatinine clearance [7] have as well been suggested to increase risk of fistula formation.

Protective patient related factors: Neoadjuvant chemoradiation, which may reduce exocrine pancreatic secretion, and diabetes mellitus, have been reported to decrease fistula incidence. [8]

Disease Related Risk Factors

Pancreatic parenchyma consistency: A soft pancreatic stump has been related to higher risk of fistula formation. Soft texture is characterized by the absence of fibrosis and the presence of pancreatic edema and inflammatory cell infiltration. Such traits make the anastomosis more difficult to perform and therefore more prone to fail. Pancreatic resection for chronic pancreatitis or obstructive pancreatic carcinoma is hence less likely to become complicated by fistula development. [9]

Pancreatic duct caliber: An association between a Wirsung's duct caliber equal to or under 3 mm and fistula formation has been described. A reduced duct diameter complicates the achievement of the pancreatic-enteric anastomosis [10, 11].

Other disease related risk factors: Increased pancreatic juice secretion and pathologic diagnosis (distal cholangiocarcinoma, benign islet tumors, intraductal papillary mucinous neoplasia, ampullary or duodenal carcinoma, pancreatic cystadenomas, duodenal adenomas) have also been associated with pancreatic fistula [6, 12].

Surgical Risk Factors

Intraoperative blood loss: High volume intraoperative blood loss is an important factor that predisposes to anastomotic failure and fistula formation. Yeh et al. proposed that a loss of over 1500 ml entailed a higher chance of fistula development [7].

Invagination anatomosis: Three different methods have been employed to complete pancreaticojejunostomy. Duct-to-mucosa anastomosis requires sewing the pancreatic duct directly to the intestinal mucosa. Invagination techniques (end-to-end or end-to-side) entail incorporating both the duct and the serosal layer into the bowel. A randomized trail found lower fistula rates to be associated with invagination techniques [13], although additional studies are required to confirm this benefit.

Surgical procedures that entail no demonstrated benefit: There are no conclusive data supporting the employment of stents across the pancreaticojejunal anastomosis. Studies have produced conflicting results [5, 14, 15]. This technique is however utilized by some groups in selected patients. Pancreaticogastrostomy has been evaluated as an alternative to pancreaticojejunostomy. The low gastric pH partially prevents the activation of pancreatic enzymes, providing theoretical support for the first approach. Although pancreaticogastrostomy is currently considered an acceptable alternative to the classic method, it has however failed to demonstrate a benefit in fistula development rates. A randomized trail found comparable outcomes regarding fistulae in both procedures [16].

Risk Factors for Distal Pancreatectomy

Complications of distal pancreatectomy have been considerably less thoroughly investigated. Pancreatic body transection and the absence of duct ligation are the two most reliably identified risk factors [17]. Other suggested risk factors are soft pancreatic tissue, spleen-preserving procedures, and the lack of postoperative prophylactic octreotide [18], but further study is required before their clinical relevance may be determined [3].

Most Relevant Risk Factors

Of all the mentioned factors, soft pancreatic parenchyma, high volume surgical blood loss, low caliber pancreatic duct and duodenal, cystic, ampullary and islet cell pathology are the conditions that entail a higher risk for the development of pancreatic fistulae [3].

Clinical Manifestations

Symptoms vary depending on the anatomic structures affected by a fistula, as well as on its size. Pancreatic fistula can be a serious, potentially fatal complication, but also a benign process with no clinical consequences.

External Fistulae

External fistulae imply the contact of pancreatic fluid with the skin, which may lead to skin excoriation and infection. They are also associated with electrolyte imbalance and malnutrition, as well as bleeding.

Internal Fistulae

Internal fistulae may cause the formation of abdominal collections (pseudocysts), which may in turn become infected, producing abdominal pain and fever. If a vessel is comprised in a pseudocyst, its walls can become eroded by the enzyme-rich fluid, resulting in pseudoaneurysm and subsequent intraabdominal bleeding, a potentially fatal complication.

If the secreted fluid is not contained by the structures surrounding the pancreatic gland, pancreatic ascites may appear, which may in turn produce abdominal distention, a variable intensity of abdominal pain, anorexia, malnutrition and asthenia.

The capability of pancreatic secretion to erode tissues grants it the capacity to penetrate into all neighboring organs: bowel, biliary tree, portal vein, and also supradiaphragmatic structures such as the pleura, bronchial tree, mediastinum and pericardium [19]. The drainage of pancreatic fluid into each particular structure produces symptoms characteristic of those vital parts. Thoracopancreatic fistulae can trigger dyspnea, cough, dysphagia or chest pain.

All collections have the potential of becoming infected and producing sepsis.

In 2005, the ISGPF developed a clinical grading system for postoperative pancreatic fistulae [2]:

Grade A is the most common grade. It is defined as a transient fistula with no clinical impact. It requires no treatment and it does not delay patient discharge.

Grade B defines a clinically relevant fistula. It may be associated with pain, fever and leukocytosis, and usually precludes oral feeding. Drains should be left in place, and if abdominal collections are detected on CT or US, they should be repositioned. Antibiotics are usually employed and somatostatin analogues may be used. Discharge is delayed and costs are increased.

Grade C defines a fistula that requires major changes in management, results in sepsis and organ dysfunction and is potentially life threatening. Treatment should be aggressive, including admission in an intensive care unit and surgical exploration.

DIAGNOSIS

Pancreatic fistula should be suspected by its clinical manifestations. The diagnosis is supported by radiological findings, and confirmed by high amylase concentrations in the extravasated fluid.

Physical Examination

Physical findings depend on the location of the drained fluid. If a pseudocyst is formed, a palpable mass may be found. Abdominal distention, flank dullness and a tympanic central abdomen may be discovered in the setting of pancreatic ascites.

A pancreaticothoracic fistula may cause unilateral o bilateral dullness over thoracic percussion and decreased breath sounds upon auscultation on the lower thorax if pleural effusion is present. Wheezing can be detected in relation with pancreaticobronchial communications.

External fistulae can produce skin irritation accompanied by fluid oozing.

Fever, hypotension and tachycardia will be present if infection or sepsis develop.

Laboratory Findings

Routine blood counts and blood chemistry determinations are unspecific. Leukocytosis may be present in the setting of infected collections or sepsis, along with high levels of acute phase reactants (C-reactive protein (CRP), fibrinogen, ferritin, erythrocyte sedimentation rate (ESR)). Nutrition markers (cholesterol, tryglicerides, albumin, prealbumin, retinol binding protein) can be diminished. The detection of amylase rich fluid is the hallmark of pancreatic fistulae. Samples from collections, ascites or effusions, as well as externally drained fluid, should be retrieved. Amylase levels over 3 times the normal upper limit are suggestive of the diagnosis, levels over 5 times the upper limit are highly charasteristic, and levels over 4000 U/L along with 2.5 to 3 g/dL of albumin concentration are frequently ascertained.

Imaging Tests

Magnetic resonance cholangiopancreatography (MRCP), endoscopic retrograde cholangiopancreatography (ERCP), fistulography and computerized tomography (CT) are the most useful radiological tests for the diagnosis of pancreatic fistulae.

MRCP is regarded as the initial diagnostic tool [20], and secretine-induced pancreatic ductal secretion, which results in filling and dilation of the pancreatic duct, has proved itself valuable in the identification of pancreatic fistulae when secretine is administered at the time of performing MRCP [21]. Its noninvasive, dynamic nature, along with the possibility of obtaining axial images, make it a safer and superior source of information compared to ERCP, whose diagnostic failure regarding pancreatic fistulae has been estimated in as high as 25 percent. *ERCP* should be performed when MRCP is not diagnostic and a high clinical suspicion persists, and also if endoscopic therapeutic maneuvers are required or anticipated (Figures 1 and 2). Its invasive nature, not devoid of a considerable risk of serious complications, accounts for its main drawback.

Fistolography may demonstrate the location of the internal communication of an external fistula, as well as help repositioning catheters to improve drainage when these are present.

CT is useful in demonstrating collections.

Ultrasound endoscopy has been also described as a useful tool in the diagnostic workup of pancreatic fistulae in a case in which MRCP did not reach the diagnosis [22].

TREATMENT

Conservative Treatment

The initial management of pancreatic fistulae must be conservative, regardless of the point drainage, for 75 percent of them resolve without invasive therapies.

Patients should be made nil per os (NPO) and provided with nutritional support to correct malnutrition. Nasojejunal feeding is favored over parenteral nutrition, for it avoids the risk of catheter infection, diminishes costs and has been associated with higher closure rates than the latter [23].

Antibiotics are given prophylactically or if signs of infection are present, and adjusted according to information from cultures [3]. Electrolyte disturbances must be corrected through fluid hydration. Adequate skin care should be provided to prevent or treat excoriations.

Treatment with somatostanin analogues is considered controversial. Some studies have found that such drugs are able to reduce fistula output [24], whereas others have not demonstrated a benefit [25], and direct clinical benefit has not been proven. Authors are thus divided regarding its use [1, 9] and no clear recommendation can be made. Somatostatin analogues should probably be considered in high-output fistulae.

Endoscopic Therapy

Endoscopic treatment should be the next step if fistula closure is not achieved after a few weeks of conservative treatment. This approach is less commonly used in postoperative pancreatic fistulae. Endoscopic techniques are aimed at draining abdominal fluid collections, achieving dilation of strictures and relieving excessive intraductal pressure.

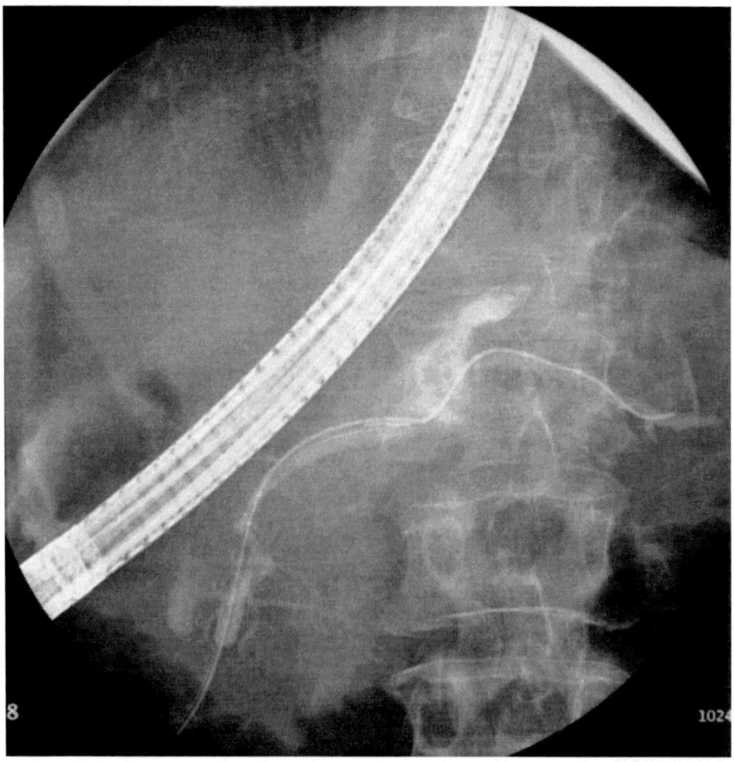

Figure 2. ERCP image showing guidewire progression into the caudal portion of Wirsung's duct, which contains contrast fluid as well. Contrast fluid may be also observed in the fistula.

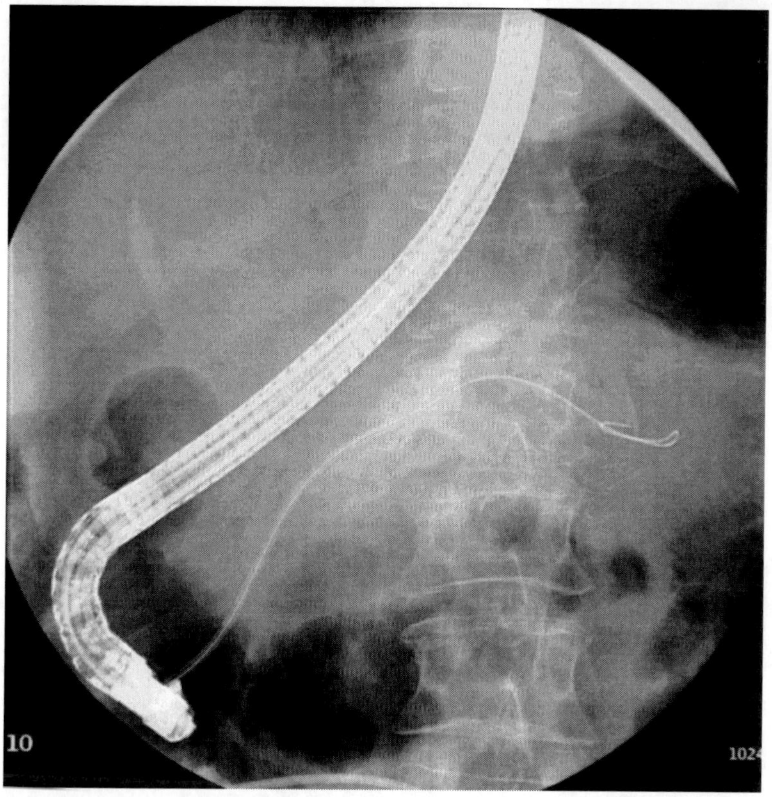

Figure 3. ERCP image showing the introduction of a plastic pancreatic stent aiming to achieve disruption bridging. Contrast fluid is still present in the fistula.

The latter maneuver is accomplished by either placing a stent across the duodenal papilla or by bridging whatever ductal disruptions may be present. The second procedure is supported by the idea that the lower resistance path created in that manner should produce the fluid to flow in an antegrade direction instead of through the fistula, consequently facilitating fistula clousure.

The usefulness of disruption bridging has not been definitively demonstrated [26, 27], but it is recommended by some authors (Figures 3 and 4).

A success rate of 85 percent has been reported after treatment with endoscopic methods [28], which should, however, be only performed at highly experienced centers.

Potential complications include stent occlusion, stent migration, duodenal erosion or perforation, acute pancreatitis, and infection. Prophylactic antibitotics are usually administered before the procedure.

Radiological Therapy

Percutaneous radiological procedures are mainly recommended in external or postoperative fistulae. Percutaneous drainage of an internal fistula entails the risk of secondary development of an external fistula, and should thus be contemplated only after conservative, endoscopic or surgical approaches have failed or are contraindicated.

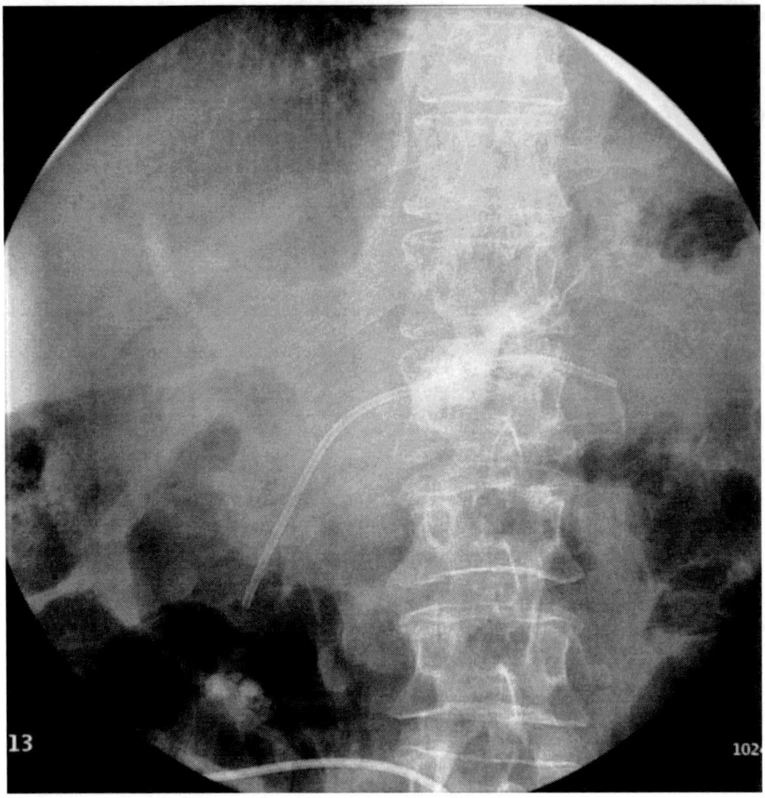

Figure 4. ERCP image showing definitive location of a plastic pancreatic stent after achievement of pancreatic duct disruption bridging. Contrast fluid remains inside the pancreatic fistula.

Percutaneous drainage of collections, either through catheter repositioning or percutaneous radiological treatment, is part of the therapeutic range defined by the ISGPF for grade B fistulae. Evacuation of postoperative collections after pancreatic resection is the primary role of percutaneous approaches, which achieve fistula resolution frequently over three to six weeks, allowing reoperation of postoperative pancreatic leaks to be avoided in a considerable proportion of patients. Radiologic management of chronic external fistulae, either surgical or of other etiology in origin, has not been adequately established. Successful outcomes after drainage with catheters [29] and percutaneous embolization [30] have been reported.

Surgical Treatment

Surgical intervention is the option of choice in the treatment of chronic fistulae when other approaches fail. Three to six months are generally waited in order to permit the development of a fibrotic tract, and detailed characterization of the fistula by imaging tests should be obtained.

Surgical management is part of the therapeutic range defined by the ISGPF for grade C fistulae, which includes patients with a deteriorating clinical status, evidence of sepsis, or organ dysfunction.

Proposed options to treat such situations include [9]:

- Placement of abundant peripancreatic drainage with the intention to repair the site of leakage.
- Transformation of the pancreatic anastomosis into another type of anastomosis (e.g., conversion of a pancreaticojejunostomy to a pancreaticogastrostomy or vice versa).
- Completion pancreatectomy.

It must be however kept in mind that these complex interventions entail very high risk when performed on a severely ill patient. Resection of a few centimeters of the pancreatic stump and completion of a new anastomosis (pancreatic-enteric or pancreatic-gastric) or total pancreatectomy may culminate in abscess formation, sepsis, or anastomotic failure, with very high subsequent mortality [2, 31, 32].

Reintervention should hence be an infrequent event, for most postoperative pancreatic fistulae respond favorably to noninvasive therapy.

Acute, non postoperative pancreatic fistulae may be controlled by oversewing of the anatomic disruption.

Chronic external fistulae may be effectively treated by enteric drainage, although this approach is associated with fistula recurrence [33]. Different approaches for the treatment of this complication have been reported. The choice of the technique is made after consideration of factors such as the location of the disruption, status of the pancreatic remnant upstream from the ductal disruption, prior interventions and presence of vascular thrombosis or necrosis.

Left pancreatic resection with splenic conservation (for leaks originating in the body or tail), Roux-en-Y pancreaticojejunostomy, Roux-en-Y cystojejunostomy and Roux-en-Y fistulojejunostomy have all been described as potentially effective treatments for chronic external fistulae, with an overall success rate of 90 percent and a mortality of 6 percent [33]. When performing fistulojejunostomy, the anastomosis must be accomplished close to the gland, since obliteration of the fistula tract over time may produce therapeutical failure.

Fibrin Glue

N-butyl-2-cyanoacrylate is a stable monomer in liquid state that polymerizes into a solid on contact with body fluids at neutral pH.

Fibrin glue was employed with success in postoperative fistulae which appeared after drain removal in a report [34]. The substance was injected into the fistula tract and resulted in fistula resolution in a high proportion of patients, especially in the group affected by low output fistulae.

N-butyl-2-cyanoacrylate was also used in a pilot study that included internal and external fistulae in 12 patients unfit for surgery due to comorbidity. The glue was delivered to the location of the leak utilizing endoscopes until sealing was attained. Success in 8 patients was described [35].

PREVENTION

Several strategies have been evaluated to prevent postoperative formation of pancreatic fistulae, with variable success.

Technical Modifications

Pancreatic remnant reconstruction variations: Classic Whipple procedure traditionally uses pancreaticojejunostomy for reconstruction of the pancreatic-enteric communication. This method connects the remaining pancreatic tissue to a loop of jejunum, a logical decision due to the rich blood supply and mobile mesentery present in this bowel segment.

However, fistula development rates of 10 percent in average [36] have been consistently reported. Pancreticogastrostomy, which is accomplished by anastomosing the pancreas to the posterior gastric wall, has emerged as an acceptable alternative to the classical approach. Gastric anastomosis has three potential advantages: the thickness of the gastric wall and its rich blood supply favor anastomotic healing; the location of the stomach, anatomically close to the pancreatic gland, permits a tension free anastomosis; and as previously mentioned, the low gastric pH prevents complete pancreatic enzyme activation and subsequent anastomotic damage. However, as mentioned above, these theoretical benefits have not been reflected in diminished fistula formation rates [16]. Pancreaticogastrostomy is currently considered a reasonable alternative to pancreticojejunostomy, but it does not provide a benefit by means of decreased fistula formation.

Variations to the pancreaticojejunostomy: As mentioned above a randomized trail found lower fistula rates to be associated with invagination techniques [13] compared to duct to mucosa anastomoses. More studies are needed to confirm these results.

Stent placement across pancreaticojejunostomy: This approach is sustained by the argument that stent placement protects the pancreatic duct from iatrogenic injury and facilitates a more precise placement of sutures during the duct-to-mucosa anastomosis.

Studies evaluating this technique produced conflicting results, and reports describing decreased rates of pancreatic fistula have been as numerous as those finding no benefit or even potential harm with routine use of stent placement [5, 14, 15]. Some authors implement stenting when the pancreatic duct is less than or equal to 3 mm in diameter [37].

Use of separate jejunal limbs for pancreatic and biliary anastomosis: This technique is advocated by some surgeons [38], on the basis that the addition of a Roux loop may limit activation of pancreatic enzymes by biliary secretions, which often occurs when a single loop is used. This approach is yet to be proven by studies that render quality evidence.

Distal pancreatectomy: preventive measures include pancreatic duct ligation, staple versus suture closure of the stump and fibrin glue sealing of the pancreatic remnant. A study that described the outcomes of 126 distal pancreatectomies found successful ligation of the main pancreatic duct to be significantly associated with a decrease of fistula rates when compared to no ligation (9.6 percent versus 34.5 percent) [39].

A subsequent meta-analysis demonstrated no significant difference between handsewn and stapler closure of the pancreatic remnant [40]. Fibrin glue has been reported to decrease pancreatic fistula rates when applied to the sectioned end of the pancreatic duct in distal pancreatectomy. These results have been nevertheless criticized for high selection bias [3].

Prophylactic Somatostatin and Its Analogues

Somatostatin and its analogues (octreotide, vapreotide, lanreotide) inhibit the secretion of secretin, glucose dependent insulinotropic peptide, cholecystokinin, insulin, vasoactive intestinal polypeptide, and glucagon, thus inactivating gastric and pancreatic exocrine secretion. The use of somatostatin and its analogues also renders a hardening of the pancreatic parenchyma, and is capable of facilitating the performance of pancreatic-enteric anastomosis. Prophylactic somatostatin or its analogues may be administered preoperatively and/or intraoperatively during pancreatic resection.

Published reports regarding the utility of this therapy vary widely in the agent used, method of administration, definitions of complications, and the evaluated outcomes, especially concerning pancreatic fistula definition. These circumstances make comparisons and conclusion drawing difficult.

A meta-analysis of ten randomized trials evaluating patients undergoing pancreatic resection performed by different techniques with a high gathered n (n=1918), in which the use of somatostatin or its analogues was compared with a control group, found the following results [41]: there was no reduction in mortality; overall morbidity was significantly reduced (OR 0.62); specific pancreatic complications (fistulae, anastomotic leaks, intra-abdominal collections or abscesses) were significantly reduced (OR 0.45), with the greatest benefit being observed in resections motivated by neoplasia; there was no significant reduction of pancreas-related complications after pancreaticoduodenectomy or distal pancreatectomy.

A subsequent retrospective analysis evaluated the effect of prophylactic ocrcotide in a series of patients. Patients were classified following the International Study Group on Pancreatic Fistula (ISGPF) grading system. Groups were formed according to the presence or absence of one or more risk factors for the development of pancreatic fistula (pancreatic duct equal to or less than 3 mm in diameter, soft pancreatic parenchyma, ampullary, duodenal, cystic or islet cell pathology or intraoperative blood loss greater than 1,000 mL). Ocreotide use did not prove itself beneficial when administered to all patients regarding pancreatic fistula rates, other non-fistulous complications and hospitalization duration and costs. Octreotide did, however, offer a benefit when administered selectively to patients with at least one risk factor for fistula development. Such patients were less likely to develop clinically relevant fistulae (ISGPF grades B and C) when prophylactically treated with octreotide compared to the ones who received no prophylaxis. The authors justified their observations by the fact that the presence of risk factors increases the incidence of all fistula grades, that fistulae in the setting of low risk glands tend to present grade A characteristics (clinically irrelevant), whereas in high risk glands B/C grades are more frequent, and that octreotide administration in patients with risk factors probably reduces the ratio of clinical relevant fistulae to biochemical fistulae. The authors suggest prophylactic octreotide use in pancreatic resection performed on patients with risk factors for the development of pancreatic fistula [3].

A subsequent meta-analysis compiling the data from eight randomized controlled trials that evaluated outcomes of pancreaticoduodenectomy failed to demonstrate differences in postoperative morbidity and mortality rates [42]. A randomized trial examining octreotide in distal pancreatectomy did not support prophylactic administration [43].

Because of the divergent results a firm recommendation regarding the use of prophylactic somatostatin or its analogues in patients undergoing pancreatic resection cannot be made. Their administration may be reasonable in patients who present risk factors for the development of fistulae, but this should be confirmed in further studies.

REFERENCES

[1] Mahvi, D. Defining, controlling, and treating a pancreatic fistula. *J. Gastrointest. Surg.* 2009;13:1187-8.

[2] Bassi, C., Dervenis, C., Butturini, G., Fingerhut, A., Yeo, C., Izbicki, J., Neoptolemos, J., Sarr, M., Traverso, W., Buchler, M. Postoperative pancreatic fistula: an international study group (ISGPF) definition. *Surgery* 2005;138:8-13.

[3] Callery, M. P., Pratt, W. B., Vollmer, C. M., Jr. Prevention and management of pancreatic fistula. *J. Gastrointest. Surg.* 2009;13:163-73.

[4] Kaman, L., Behera, A., Singh, R., Katariya, R. N. Internal pancreatic fistulas with pancreatic ascites and pancreatic pleural effusions: recognition and management. *ANZ J. Surg.* 2001;71:221-5.

[5] Matsusue, S., Takeda, H., Nakamura, Y., Nishimura, S., Koizumi, S. A prospective analysis of the factors influencing pancreaticojejunostomy performed using a single method, in 100 consecutive pancreaticoduodenectomies. *Surg. Today* 1998;28:719-26.

[6] Lin, J. W., Cameron, J. L., Yeo, C. J., Riall, T. S., Lillemoe, K. D. Risk factors and outcomes in postpancreaticoduodenectomy pancreaticocutaneous fistula. *J. Gastrointest. Surg.* 2004;8:951-9.

[7] Yeh, T. S., Jan, Y. Y., Jeng, L. B., Hwang, T. L., Wang, C. S., Chen, S. C., Chao, T. C., Chen, M. F. Pancreaticojejunal anastomotic leak after pancreaticoduodenectomy--multivariate analysis of perioperative risk factors. *J. Surg. Res.* 1997;67:119-25.

[8] Ishikawa, O., Ohigashi, H., Imaoka, S., Teshima, T., Inoue, T., Sasaki, Y., Iwanaga, T., Nakaizumi, A. Concomitant benefit of preoperative irradiation in preventing pancreas fistula formation after pancreatoduodenectomy. *Arch. Surg.* 1991;126:885-9.

[9] Butturini, G., Daskalaki, D., Molinari, E., Scopelliti, F., Casarotto, A., Bassi, C. Pancreatic fistula: definition and current problems. *J. Hepatobiliary Pancreat. Surg.* 2008;15:247-51.

[10] Muscari, F., Suc, B., Kirzin, S., Hay, J. M., Fourtanier, G., Fingerhut, A., Sastre, B., Chipponi, J., Fagniez, P. L., Radovanovic, A. Risk factors for mortality and intra-abdominal complications after pancreatoduodenectomy: multivariate analysis in 300 patients. *Surgery* 2006;139:591-8.

[11] Lermite, E., Pessaux, P., Brehant, O., Teyssedou, C., Pelletier, I., Etienne, S., Arnaud, J. P. Risk factors of pancreatic fistula and delayed gastric emptying after pancreaticoduodenectomy with pancreaticogastrostomy. *J. Am. Coll. Surg.* 2007;204:588-96.

[12] Poon, R. T., Lo, S. H., Fong, D., Fan, S. T., Wong, J. Prevention of pancreatic anastomotic leakage after pancreaticoduodenectomy. *Am. J. Surg.* 2002;183:42-52.

[13] Berger, A. C., Howard, T. J., Kennedy, E. P., Sauter, P. K., Bower-Cherry, M., Dutkevitch, S., Hyslop, T., Schmidt, C. M., Rosato, E. L., Lavu, H., Nakeeb, A., Pitt, H. A., Lillemoe, K. D., Yeo, C. J. Does type of pancreaticojejunostomy after pancreaticoduodenectomy decrease rate of pancreatic fistula? A randomized, prospective, dual-institution trial. *J. Am. Coll. Surg*. 2009;208:738-47; discussion 747-9.

[14] Roder, J. D., Stein, H. J., Bottcher, K. A., Busch, R., Heidecke, C. D., Siewert, J. R. Stented versus nonstented pancreaticojejunostomy after pancreatoduodenectomy: a prospective study. *Ann. Surg*. 1999;229:41-8.

[15] Bartoli, F. G., Arnone, G. B., Ravera, G., Bachi, V. Pancreatic fistula and relative mortality in malignant disease after pancreaticoduodenectomy. Review and statistical meta-analysis regarding 15 years of literature. *Anticancer Res*. 1991;11:1831-48.

[16] Yeo, C. J., Cameron, J. L., Maher, M. M., Sauter, P. K., Zahurak, M. L., Talamini, M. A., Lillemoe, K. D., Pitt, H. A. A prospective randomized trial of pancreaticogastrostomy versus pancreaticojejunostomy after pancreaticoduodenectomy. *Ann. Surg*. 1995;222:580-8; discussion 588-92.

[17] Pannegeon, V., Pessaux, P., Sauvanet, A., Vullierme, M. P., Kianmanesh, R., Belghiti, J. Pancreatic fistula after distal pancreatectomy: predictive risk factors and value of conservative treatment. *Arch. Surg*. 2006;141:1071-6; discussion 1076.

[18] Ridolfini, M. P., Alfieri, S., Gourgiotis, S., Di Miceli, D., Rotondi, F., Quero, G., Manghi, R., Doglietto, G. B. Risk factors associated with pancreatic fistula after distal pancreatectomy, which technique of pancreatic stump closure is more beneficial? *World J. Gastroenterol*. 2007;13:5096-100.

[19] Fulcher, A. S., Capps, G. W., Turner, M. A. Thoracopancreatic fistula: clinical and imaging findings. *J. Comput. Assist. Tomogr*. 1999;23:181-7.

[20] Vyas, S., Gogoi, D., Sinha, S. K., Singh, P., Yadav, T. D., Khandelwal, N. Pancreaticopleural fistula: an unusual complication of pancreatitis diagnosed with magnetic resonance cholangiopancreatography. *Jop* 2009;10:671-3.

[21] Alkaade, S., Fattahi, R., Balci, N. C., Akduman, E. I., Garvin, P. J., Modanlou, K. A., Burton, F. R. Acute pancreatic graft fistula and peripancreatic fluid collection: demonstration by secretin-stimulated MRI. *Magn. Reson. Imaging* 2009;27:1005-8.

[22] Kutz Leoz, M. IGR, Vila Costas, J. J., Martínez Echeverría, A., Elizalde Apestegui, I., Basterra Ederra, M., Gómez Alonso, M., Zozaya Urmeneta, J. M. Pleural efusión secondary to pancreaticopleural fistula following acute pancreatitis. *Gastroenterol. Hepatol*. 2012 Feb;35:70-3.

[23] Klek, S., Sierzega, M., Turczynowski, L., Szybinski, P., Szczepanek, K., Kulig, J. Enteral and parenteral nutrition in the conservative treatment of pancreatic fistula: a randomized clinical trial. *Gastroenterology*; 141: 157-63, 163 e1.

[24] Gayral, F., Campion, J. P., Regimbeau, J. M., Blumberg, J., Maisonobe, P., Topart, P., Wind, P. Randomized, placebo-controlled, double-blind study of the efficacy of lanreotide 30 mg PR in the treatment of pancreatic and enterocutaneous fistulae. *Ann. Surg*. 2009;250:872-7.

[25] Sancho, J. J., di Costanzo, J., Nubiola, P., Larrad, A., Beguiristain, A., Roqueta, F., Franch, G., Oliva, A., Gubern, J. M., Sitges-Serra, A. Randomized double-blind placebo-controlled trial of early octreotide in patients with postoperative enterocutaneous fistula. *Br. J. Surg*. 1995;82:638-41.

[26] Bracher, G. A., Manocha, A. P., DeBanto, J. R., Gates, L. K., Jr., Slivka, A., Whitcomb, D. C., Bleau, B. L., Ulrich, C. D., 2nd, Martin, S. P. Endoscopic pancreatic duct stenting to treat pancreatic ascites. *Gastrointest. Endosc*. 1999;49:710-5.

[27] Telford, J. J., Farrell, J. J., Saltzman, J. R., Shields, S. J., Banks, P. A., Lichtenstein, D. R., Johannes, R. S., Kelsey, P. B., Carr-Locke, D. L. Pancreatic stent placement for duct disruption. *Gastrointest. Endosc*. 2002;56:18-24.

[28] Alexakis, N., Sutton, R., Neoptolemos, J. P. Surgical treatment of pancreatic fistula. *Dig. Surg*. 2004;21:262-74.

[29] Cabay, J. E., Boverie, J. H., Dondelinger, R. F. Percutaneous catheter drainage of external fistulas of the pancreatic ducts. *Eur. Radiol*. 1998;8:445-8.

[30] Hirota, M., Kamekawa, K., Tashima, T., Mizumoto, M., Ohara, C., Beppu, T., Shimada, S., Yamaguchi, Y., Ogawa, M. Percutaneous embolization of the distal pancreatic duct to treat intractable pancreatic juice fistula. *Pancreas* 2001;22:214-6.

[31] Aranha, G. V., Aaron, J. M., Shoup, M., Pickleman, J. Current management of pancreatic fistula after pancreaticoduodenectomy. *Surgery* 2006;140:561-8; discussion 568-9.

[32] Munoz-Bongrand, N., Sauvanet, A., Denys, A., Sibert, A., Vilgrain, V., Belghiti, J. Conservative management of pancreatic fistula after pancreaticoduodenectomy with pancreaticogastrostomy. *J. Am. Coll. Surg*. 2004;199:198-203.

[33] Voss, M., Ali, A., Eubanks, W. S., Pappas, T. N. Surgical management of pancreaticocutaneous fistula. *J. Gastrointest. Surg*. 2003;7:542-6.

[34] Cothren, C. C., McIntyre, R. C., Jr., Johnson, S., Stiegmann, G. V. Management of low-output pancreatic fistulas with fibrin glue. *Am. J. Surg*. 2004;188:89-91.

[35] Seewald, S., Brand, B., Groth, S., Omar, S., Mendoza, G., Seitz, U., Yasuda, I., Xikun, H., Nam, V. C., Xu, H., Thonke, F., Soehendra, N. Endoscopic sealing of pancreatic fistula by using N-butyl-2-cyanoacrylate. *Gastrointest. Endosc*. 2004;59:463-70.

[36] Strasberg, S. M., Drebin, J. A., Soper, N. J. Evolution and current status of the Whipple procedure: an update for gastroenterologists. *Gastroenterology* 1997;113:983-94.

[37] Pratt, W. B., Callery, M. P., Vollmer, C. M., Jr. Risk prediction for development of pancreatic fistula using the ISGPF classification scheme. *World J. Surg*. 2008;32:419-28.

[38] Sikora, S. S., Posner, M. C. Management of the pancreatic stump following pancreaticoduodenectomy. *Br. J. Surg*. 1995;82:1590-7.

[39] Bilimoria, M. M., Cormier, J. N., Mun, Y., Lee, J. E., Evans, D. B., Pisters, P. W. Pancreatic leak after left pancreatectomy is reduced following main pancreatic duct ligation. *Br. J. Surg*. 2003;90:190-6.

[40] Knaebel, H. P., Diener, M. K., Wente, M. N., Buchler, M. W., Seiler, C. M. Systematic review and meta-analysis of technique for closure of the pancreatic remnant after distal pancreatectomy. *Br. J. Surg*. 2005;92:539-46.

[41] Connor, S., Alexakis, N., Garden, O. J., Leandros, E., Bramis, J., Wigmore, S. J. Meta-analysis of the value of somatostatin and its analogues in reducing complications associated with pancreatic surgery. *Br. J. Surg*. 2005;92:1059-67.

[42] Zeng, Q., Zhang, Q., Han, S., Yu, Z., Zheng, M., Zhou, M., Bai, J., Jin, R. Efficacy of somatostatin and its analogues in prevention of postoperative complications after pancreaticoduodenectomy: a meta-analysis of randomized controlled trials. *Pancreas* 2008;36:18-25.

[43] Suc, B., Msika, S., Piccinini, M., Fourtanier, G., Hay, J. M., Flamant, Y., Fingerhut, A., Fagniez, P. L., Chipponi, J. Octreotide in the prevention of intra-abdominal complications following elective pancreatic resection: a prospective, multicenter randomized controlled trial. *Arch. Surg*. 2004;139:288-94; discussion 295.

In: Fistuals and Fissures
Editors: Dmitri Pavlovich and Sergei Ivanovich

ISBN: 978-1-62618-068-0

Chapter 6

DIALYSIS ACCESS-ASSOCIATED STEAL SYNDROME

Huai-Min Chen and Ying-Fu Chen*

Division of Cardiovascular Surgery, Department of Surgery,
Kaohsiung Medical University Hospital, Kaohsiung, Taiwan
Graduate Institute of Medicine, College of Medicine, Kaohsiung Medical University,
Kaohsiung, Taiwan

ABSTRACT

The steal phenomenon is a rarely seen multifactorial complication after hemodialysis access creation. The clinical pictures of steal are variants from mild pain or coldness of distal hand (stage I) to severe tissue necrosis or gangrene (stage IV). The reported incidence ranges from 1.6% to 11%. The occurrences are higher in patients with distal prosthetic graft, side-to-side anastomosis of AV fistula, Diabeties Mellitus, hypertension, coronary artery disease, and female gender. The diagnosis is largely based on the clinical presentations but a varety of methods have been used to confirm the ischemic steal, which include color duplex ultrasound, digital photoplethysmography, pulse oxymetry, and even the infrared thermography. When the steal is suspected, an urgent vascular evaluation and prompt revision of treatment are of the essence. The pathophysiologies of steal syndrome are also various including too large shunting, increased vascular resistance peripheral to the fistula, inflow stenosis, and distal arteriopathy. The goal of treatment is to restore the distal perfusion and to maintain the access function. Many procedures are reported in the literature including access ligation, banding, correction of the inflow lesion, proximalization of arterial inflow (PAI), revision using distal inflow (RUDI), distal revascularization with interval ligation (DRIL), banding between dialysis puncture sites, minimally invasive limited ligation endoluminal-assisted revision (MILLER) banding procedure, ulnar artery dilation, transcatheter collateral veins coil embolization, and ligation of the perforating vein. Because different pathophysiologies present in different patients, we discuss and compare the many interventional strategies based on conditions of the proximal arterial stenosis, distal arterial stenosis, low-flow steal syndrome, high-flow steal syndrome, and individual specific situation.

* Corresponding author: Ying-Fu Chen MD, PhD. E-mail: yfchen@cc.kmu.edu.tw.

INTRODUCTION

Dialysis-associated steal syndrome (DASS) is a rare but challenging complication. The incidence is reported to range from 2% to 10-20% in AVF (Arterial-Venous Fistula) or AVG (Arterial-Venous Graft) [1, 2, 3]. One percent distal forearm AVF and 3-6% brachial arterial AVF/AVG with steal are required treatment [4]. Some patients experienced improvement of steal after formation of collateral circulation and the distal vessels dilation.

The time period between access creation and development of symptoms can vary from immediately to after years. If the symptoms occur acutely (in 30 days) they are mostly self-limiting and resolve with observation. On the other hand, if the symptoms occur late (>30 days), they are frequently progressive and demand more aggressive attention and treatment.

The clinical presentations range from mild symptoms such as hand pain, and coldness to more severe such as digital gangrene and tissue necrosis. With regard to gender difference, the steal is more common in female (34%) than in male (2.5%) [5], and the mean age with steal ranges from 57 years old to 61 years old [6]. The majority of patients with steal also suffered from DM (66%, 78%, and 81% in three largest reports) [7, 8, 9].

In cases of mild steal, observation is suggested because most will reverse the clinical picture in a few weeks. Some patients experienced symptoms during the course of hemodialysis because of a drop of systolic BP and even the cardiac output. In this situation, management is simply to withdraw the antihypertensive medications on the day of hemodialysis.

Rocha et al., [2] tried to determine the predictors of steal syndrome in hemodialysis patients, and they enumerate the correlations between steal and DM (P=0.002), brachiomedian fistula (P=0.016), and side-to-side anastomosis (P=0.003) in univariate analysis. However, in multivariate analysis, the presence of DM, side-to-side anastomosis, and female gender were found to be the independent risk factors. In comparison between the upper arm AVF and the forearm AVF, the incidence of steal in brachiocephalic and brachiobasilic fistula is about 10-25%, in the forearm prosthetic AVF it is about 4.3-6%, and in radiocephalic AVF it is 1-1.8% [10], so some authors suggested that after failure of radiocephalic fistula, proximal radial or ulnar-based AV (arterial-venous) access can be performed to prevent the steal caused by the brachial-based AV access. The long-term patency of the AV access based on the proximal radial or ulnar arteries has been proved. In radiocephalic fistula, retrograde flow in the radial artery toward the proximal occurs in about 70% of patients [11], the majority of whom are asymptomatic. However, if the collateral blood flow from the ulnar artery is inadequate, ischemia will present, and in more serious cases with proximal artery stenosis or occlusion, ischemia will be severe.

PATHOPHYSIOLOGY

After access creation, the imbalance between low-resistance outflow of AV access and high-resistance outflow of arterial system will present, and then the blood is shunted through the AV access to low-resistance venous system. The normal response is significant increasing compensatory blood flow through the outflow artery which causes the dilation of donor artery and even the autogenous vein of AV access. Such vessel dilation is mediated by the NO release of endothelial cells in response to the high blood flow [12].

The physiological steal occurs in about 70% of radiocephalic fistulas and about 90% of brachial artery fistulas [2, 13] but symptoms of hand ischemia only occur in 1-2% of distal fistula and 5-10 times of brachial arterial fistulas [3], but the etiology and mechanism is different from lower limb ischemia caused by peripheral arterial disease (PAD).

The diameter of inflow artery is a key point to determine the blood flow through the access. In radiocephalic AVF, the blood flow may amount to 500-800 ml/min; and in axillary/brachial-based AVF the blood flow can increase to more than 2000 ml/min. The systemic finger pressure can be above 100 mmHg when the distal AVF with the blood flow is in the range of 500-800 ml/min, but the systemic finger pressure will drop to 50-60 mmHg when the elbow AVF with the blood flow increases to the range of 1500-2000 ml/min [10], so the steal is prone to occur.

Arterial Inflow Disease- Proximal Arterial Stenosis

With an etiology of steal syndrome, diagnosis and treatment are easier; the incidence of proximal stenosis in patients with ischemic hand is about 20-30%, and the incidence is less than 5% in DASS [7, 8].

Patients with proximal stenosis are prone to the comorbidities of atherosclerosis and diabetes. The locations of stenosis may present in the subclavian, axillary, or brachial artery and the detection of stenotic sites can be diagnosed by arterial duplex images, computed tomographic angiography, and catheter-directed angiography. However, a proximal stenotic lesion can be treated simply with percutaneous revascularization; in case of multiple stenosis, in-line or extra-anatomic bypass is also a choice of treatment. Combination of normal-flow access with inflow occlusion disease also leads to a worse of the ischemic condition. We can augment the inflow by interventional technique (i.e., percutaneous trasluminal angioplasty, PTA).

Patients with High-flow Access Steal

Steal syndrome in high-flow access usually involves much more complicated etiologies and treatment. High-flow ischemia is a true steal phenomenon and usually occurs in healthy vessels. The high blood flow goes through the AV access, which results in inadequate collateral flow to achieve distal tissue perfusion. If the patient suffers distal arterial stenosis or occlusion, the symptoms of steal would be more severe and significant. There is greater risk of ischemia than with normal-flow access. The ischemia is true steal in high-flow access and the blood flow is usually over 1500 to 2000 ml/min. The goal of treatment is flow reduction or bypass reconstruction.

The methods of flow reduction include banding or tapering; a small piece of Teflon or Dacron is sutured circumferentially around the access, a distance of about 2cm distal to the anastomosis is chosen, and the lumen is tightened to 4 or 5 mm. Berman et al., [7] found that if the banding achieved the relief of ischemia, thrombosis of AVF usually follows. The bypass reconstructions by which the previous AV access could be preserved are the

DRIL(Distal Revascularization with Interval Ligation), RUDI (Revision Using Distal Inflow), PAI (Proximalization of arterial inflow), and axillary loop, the results of which are similiar. These revascularization procedures are also suitable in the treatment of high-flow access steal.

Patients with Normal Flow/Low Flow Access Steal

The ischemia is usually due to the further deprivation of distal perfusion and the blood flow ranges in 500-800 ml/min. Flow reduction is not an option for patients with normal flow steal because of the high potential of thrombosis and insufficient flow of dialysis.

In the condition of normal flow steal in radiocephalic AVF, the ligation of distal radial artery is indicated because the steal can be blocked by preventing the blood come from the palmar arch after distal radial artery ligation. However, elbow brachial-based AVF the reconstruction of bypass such as the DRIL/RUDI/PAI is the optimal choice and it can achieve a success rate up to 83~100% [7, 14~18]. In patients with DM are prone to suffer the steal because lack of vascular adaptation in inflow artery and in collateral bed. Diabetic neuropathy also plays a role in sensory and motor dysfunction.

The relations of different sites AVF flow with digital pressure in patients with normal and obstructed arteries can be seen in Table 1 and 2:

Table 1. AVF flow and digital pressure in patients with normal arteries

Type of AVF	AVF flow (cc/min)	Digital pressure (mm Hg)	Risk of ischemia
Radiocephalic	500-800	>100	−
Forearm loop graft	800-130	>70	±
Brachiocephalic/basilic	1000-2000	>50	+
Axi-axilary /jugular vein	1500-2000	>70	−

Table 2. AVF flow and digital pressure in patients with obstructed arteries

Type of AVF	AVF flow (cc/min)	Digital pressure (mm Hg)	Risk of ischemia
Radiocephalic	200–255	25–35	+
Forearm loop graft	560–740	30–50	±
Brachiocephalic/basilic	600–900	20–30	++
Axil-axillary/jugular vein	750–1000	30–40	±

Reprinted permission from Tordoir et al., [10]. The two tables show the relations of different sites AVF flow with digital pressure in normal and obstructed arteries.

Clinical Stages or Grading

Stage I: Also called steal phenomenon, presence of retrograde flow but without complaints.

Stage II: Pain on exertion or during hemodialysis.

Stage III: Pain at rest.

Stage IV: Presence of ulceration/necrosis/gangrene.

DIAGNOSIS

a) By clinical pictures and physical examination:
   1. Cold fingers with a pale or blue-purple discoloration
   2. Absent or weak distal radial pulse but more prominent under manual compression of AVF
   3. Pain during HD (hemodialysis)
   4. Skin necrosis/ulceration

b) By non-invasive investigation:
   1. Blood pressure measurement (digital, wrist, elbow)
   2. Duplex ultrasonography(arteries- central and peripheral; venous- superficial and deep; collateral circulation)
   3. Transcutaneous PcO_2 measurement
   4. Waveform monitor
   5. Digital plethysmography / pulse wave recording

      If the digital pressure is less than 50mmHg or DBI (digital-brachial index) is less than 0.6 or $TcPO_2$ less than 20-30 mmHg, the steal may be found [1, 3, 10, 19].

c) Angiography from proximal to distal- it is not only used in diagnosis but also in treatment for percutaneous angioplasty.

d) Comparison the distal flow and pressure between the compression and non-compression over AVF. DBI means the ratio of digital to brachial pressure and the level less than 0.6 has the best test characteristics for steal diagnosis; the other index we can use is the systolic pressure index (SPI) which is the ratio of fistula forearm to contralateral forearm pressure, and the ideal level of SPI is 0.5-0.6 [5, 20].

Differential Diagnosis

Several conditions mimic the s/s of ischemia making diagnosis of DASS a challenge, including

- Neuropathy
- Anesthetic complications
- Peripheral nerves compression or entrapement (eg. carpal-tunnel syndrome)
- Postoperative pain and swelling
- Dystrophy and edema due to venous hypertension
- IMN(ischemic monomelic neuropathy)

The term of IMN was first reported by Wilbourn et al., in 1983 [21], but Bolton's study first described such a patient in 1979 [22]. The classic clinical pictures of IMN include an abrupt, severe irreversible motor nerve dysfunction with mild-to-moderate ischemia; and the EP(electrophysiological study) study revealed the axon-loss lesions of motor and sensory nerves. The IMN is prone to occur in patients with DM, and it usually occurred immediately after graft placement. The digital pressure indices are low but there is no critical ischemic picture.

Hye et al., [23] also disclosed that the patients with IMN usually present with underlying diabetic neuropathy and severe multifocal neuropathy under the investigation of EP study. If the patient has preexisting diabetic neuropathy, the clinical picture is more prominent after AV access creation. Although the correction of the ischemia is not related to the improvement of IMN, and permanent motor dysfunction persists, immediate correction by the AVF/AVG ligation is still mandatory.

The differences between vascular steal syndrome and ischemic monomelic neuropathy are listed in Table-3:

Table 3. Differences between Vascular Steal Syndrome VS Ischemic Monomelic Neuropathy

	Vascular Steal Syndrome	Ischemic Monomelic Neuropathy
Onset	Subtle	Abruptly
Sex	Female>Male	Female>>Male
Affected tissue	Sensory>Motor	Motor>Sensory
	(Rare in nerve)	(Diffuse axon-loss)
Ischemia	Severe	Mild
Patient character	DM>PAD/Aged	DM predominant
Underlying	Variable	Diabetic multifocal neuropathy
Location	Variable	Brachial-based access
Distal pulse	Weak-Absent	Present
Treatment	Revision	Access closure
Prognosis	Depends	Poor (in spite of treatment)

DM: diabetes mellitus; PAD: peripheral arterial disease.

The table lists the characteristic differences between vascular steal syndrome and ischemic monomelic neuropathy.

TREATMENT

The purposes of treatment are to preserve the access function and Illuminate the picture of ischemia. Before a treatment regimen is instituted, the anatomical extremities and hemodynamic access should be evaluated in detail in DASS patients. The technique of radiologic (catheter-based) intervention is considered as the first option of treatment because proximal inflow or distal outflow arterial stenosis can be managed successfully with the percutaneous angioplasty. If this procedure fails, then the surgical intervention can be the next strategy.

The timing of surgical correction for the steal is still a controversial. If no neurologic deficit exists, 80% of patients will spontaneously and significantly improve of symptoms and signs within a few weeks.

Ligation

For many diabetic patients, the most effective and the ultimate procedure to prevent the progression of ischemia and amputation is surgical ligation of the AVF, but this procedure comes at the expense of sacrificing the access and a new AVF creation in the controlateral side or in the more proximal upper extremity is required. The procedure is accepted without controversy in the condition of radiocephalic fistula with steal and the distal radial artery ligated [1, 10], prior to insuring patency of ulnar artery and palmar arch.

Banding

Banding is the most accepted as the first choice because of its simplicity, rapidity, and lower morbidity, but the traditional banding or placation causes insufficient dialysis and thrombosis or occlusion of access. The difficulty of successful banding is proper adjustment of the size to determine the required amount of stenosis. The resistance of access is increased through banding and the blood will be diverted down to the distal artery.

In cases of steal with low flow access banding is not the optimal choice [1], but in steal with high-flow access it could be considered as the initial procedure, but its disadvantages include the ineffective elimination of ischemia and the high incidence of thrombosis.

To solve the problems Shemesh et al., [24] designed a modified method in 2010. They banded the access between the dialysis puncture sites instead of banding near the anastomosis for the low-flow and high-risk steal patients. The theory is that the pressure gradient between the arterial and venous puncture sites and the high arterial flow can be maintained to support adequate blood flow which would not be possible in the procedure of traditional banding.

Table 4. Results of intraoperative digital-brachial indices

DBI	0.2	0.3	0.35	0.4	0.45	0.5	0.6	0.7
Sensitivity	0	.33	.40	.60	.80	.87	.94	.94
Specificity	.96	.88	.83	.77	.70	.64	.43	.34
PPV	0	.33	.27	.29	.30	.28	.21	.19
NPV	.86	.88	.90	.92	.97	.97	.98	.97

DBI, digital–brachial index; PPV, positive predictive value; NPV, negative predictive value.

Reprinted permission from Berman et al., [5]. The table lists the values of sensitivity, specificity, PPV, and NPV of intra-operative DBI.

The suggested criteria for high success banding include digital pressure no less than 50-60mmHg, digital/brachial pressure index no less than 0.6, and blood flow above 350 ml/min

(>400 ml/min in AVF and >600 ml/min in AVG) [24~27]. We can use the intraoperative pressure or flow monitor to achieve these banding criteria. Some authors reported that 86% of patients showed symptomatic relief and that 91% of patients achieved one-year patency rate under these criteria [25].

The sensitivity and specificity of DBI can be checked in the Table-4.

Coil Embolization

Plumb et al., [28] presented a method of transcutaneous coil embolization of distal artery to treat the steal for the patients of distal radiocephalic fistula. The authors demonstrated that if patient has multiple distal collateral arteries it is difficult to treat merely with the ligation of distal radial artery, and the method of transcutaneous coil implantation may offer a better choice and a more complete treatment. The method of embolization is not only used in artery but also can be used in the collateral veins, especially connecting with the deep vein system. More collateral vein embolizations will decrease flow stealing from the main dialysis vessel. If the flow of the AV fistula is supplied by the major collateral vein(s), then the embolization of veins is not performed [4], however, the disadvantages of venous embolization are the possibilities of coil migration to deep vein system and the subsequent formation of new collateral vessels [4].

MILLER Banding

To solve the disadvantages of insufficient flow with high thrombosis and insufficient banding with residual steal in the traditional blind banding, Miller et al., [29, 30] introduced the modified method of Minimally Invasive Limited Ligation Endoluminal-Assisted Revision (MILLER) in 2006 to treat the patients of steal syndrome or the high-flow access problems. They used the intraluminal ballon as a sizing dowel to quantify the targeted diameter during banding. The banding site is is 1-3 cm within the arterial anastomosis and is superficial enough to facilitate easy dissection. They found that the mean banding size in AVF is 4mm (2.5~6mm) and in AVG it is 3mm (3~4mm) [29]. They also suggested that the balloon sizing in steal patients should be no more than the diameter of downstream artery and that the resistance of access should increase significantly. Combination use of the nomogram [Figure 1] [30] in high-flow patients is also suggested to surgeons. The 6-months patency rate can reach 75% in steal patients and 85% in high-flow access patients, and the secondary access patency rate in 24 months also came to about 90%. The usage of intraluminal balloon sizing can also be applied in the open surgical banding procedure. Although the result is as good as revascularization procedure, some long-term potential complications may present: these include development of intimal hyperplasia after repeated balloon angioplasty and aneurismal dilatation distal to the banding site [29]. They concluded that the MILLER procedure can more readily achieve clinical success without inducing thrombosis in all access with high flow and most access with steal, though 90% of patients required rebanding to enhance clinical efficacy.

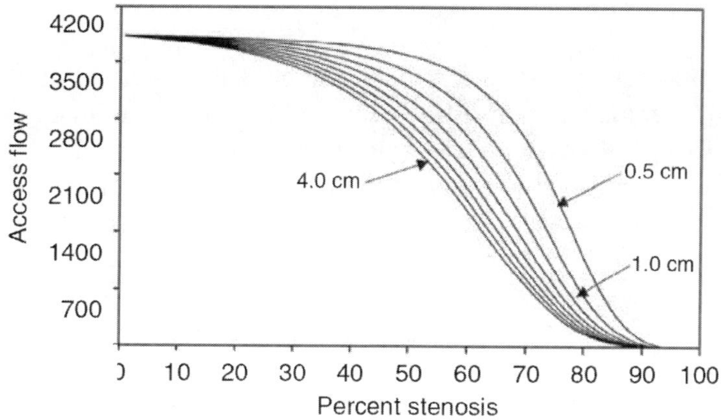

Figure 1. The curves lines represent AVF of varying diameter in the percentage of banding for reduction of total access flow.
Reprinted permission from Murray et al., [30].

Revascularization

The revascularization procedures Include DRIL, RUDI, and PAI. They are still the optimal treatments for low-flow or even normal-flow access steal. Indications of revascularization include severe pain or other symptoms which fail to ameliorate after few weeks of observation, proximal inflow disease with poor fistula flows, appearance of distal gangrene or presence of neurologic deficits, and in patients with steal or IMN. However, the limitations of revascularization depend on the vascular condition of patients, especially the distal arterial pathology. The differences between DRIL and RUDI can be seen in Figure 2.

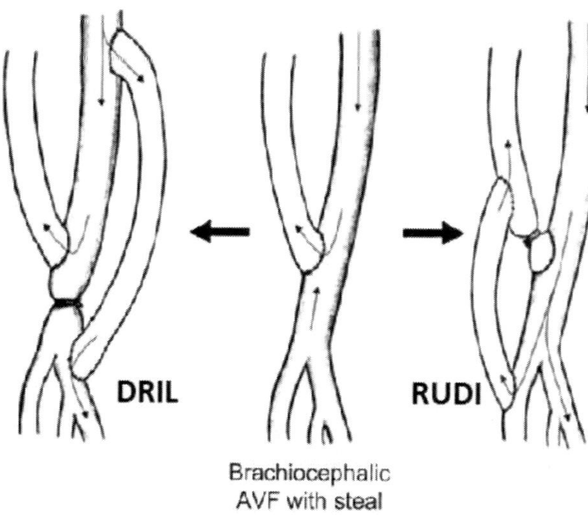

Figure 2. Reprinted permission from Berman et al., [5]. The figure demonstrates the conversions of brachio-based AVF to DRIL and RUDI.

DRIL-Distal Revascularization-Interval Ligation

The DRIL procedure was described originally by Schanzer et al., in 1988 [31]. They constructed a bypass graft (low resistance collateral) between the artery proximal to the fistula (about 5~7cm) and the artery distal to the fistula (about 3~4cm) [29, 32] and to prevent the retrograde flow from distal circulation toward to the new fistula, the native artery between the origin of AV access and distal newly bypassed anastomosis was ligated. After construction of the bypass they found that the resistance ratio between peripheral circulation and fistula was decreased; the brachial shunt fraction was decreased, also; and a great portion of blood flow toward the peripheral was noted [6]. In some patients with severe distal arterial disease, the distal revascularization alone without interval ligation may restore adequate distal perfusion [7, 33], but in patients without distal stenosis, such a procedure may deteriorate the retrograde flow and aggravate the steal condition. After ligature of the native artery, the distal blood flow depends on the graft which is a disadvantage if surgeons are concerned about severe distal ischemia following graft failure. Under such considerations, a long reversed saphenous vein graft is favored for the bypass graft, but the major problem is both the arteries and veins are usually poor in such high-risk patients.

Several study series reported the outcomes of DRIL. Huber et al., [34] demonstrated that the primary patency rate in one year was 77+-8%, three years: 74+-9%, and five years: 71+-9%; the secondary patency rate in one year was 81+-7%, three years: 76+-9%, and five years: 76+-9%, all demonstrating excellent outcomes. The wrist-brachial index (WBI) was increased from preoperative 0.46 to postoperative 0.79 (mean increased 0.34+-0.26); and the digital-brachial index (DBI) was increased from preoperative 0.25 to postoperative 0.7 (mean increased 0.41+-0.21) [34]. The success rate of symptoms relief can approach 90% with minor residual paresthesia and motor dysfunction.

In the Berman series [5, 18, 33, 35, 36] the patency in one year was 80% in AVF and 40-50% in AVG, and the four-year patency rate was also near 80% in AVF. Although the results are exciting, it is still a complex and time-consuming procedure, and the other drawback is that the distal perfusion is purely supplied and determined by the bypass graft. If the constructed graft fails, the incoming distal ischemia will be serious, so a vein graft for the interposition is recommended for the DRIL reconstruction. The distal anastomosis may also be difficult if patient has the distal arterial disease, and it is actually more morbid than banding.

RUDI- Revising Using Distal Inflow

The term RUDI has recently been addressed by Minion et al., [37] in 2005, but the technique was first described by Andrade et al., [38]. This alternate procedure which avoids the drawbacks of DRIL is ligation of the fistula at its origin and re-establishment of a bypass from distal to the brachial artery bifurcation (proximal radial or ulnar artery). In RUDI, the native artery is not ligated, so the forearm and distal hand perfusion is undisturbed and maintained, and the access length for dialysis is lengthened after the interposition graft is inserted. The length of the conduit bypass does not require a longer graft like the conduit used in DRIL (proximal about 5-7cm and distal about 3-4cm) [39]. Although the outcomes in

RUDI are similar to the DRIL, limitations also exist. If the other forearm artery is diseased or not patent, the hand ischemia would not resolve.

PAI-Proximalization of Arterial Inflow

In PAI, the previous brachial-based AV access is divided near the proximal anastomosis site and a small caliber of ePTFE graft (4-5mm) [23] is anastomosed to the venous stump of the fistula; the other end of graft is anastomsed to the more proximal brachial artery (or axillary artery) to reconstruct a new AV access. According to the study of Gradman et al [40], the brachial flow before and after PAI is better than DRIL, especially if the diameter of arterial bypass is less than 6mm [41].

The other recent study in PAI also revealed that the one-year primary and secondary patency rates were 87% and 90%, respectively [14, 42-44]. There are still limitations for the PAI procedure; it cannot be applied to loop graft fistulas and it requires patent fistula veins with good flow, and a large cohort study with long-term follow-up is lacking to make conclusive determinations.

The revascularization procedures and banding are demonstrated in the Figure 3.

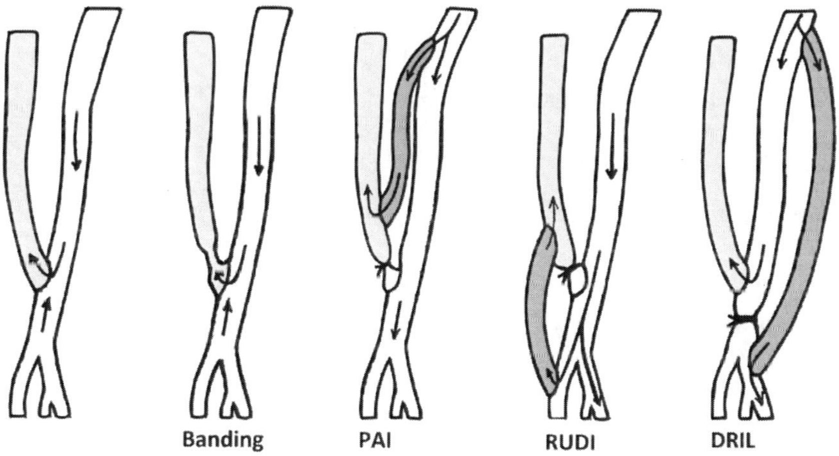

Figure 3. The all revascularization and banding procedures are demonstrated in the lined pictures. The tubes colored with dark gray indicate the interposition grafts, and the light gray ones mean the AVF(G)s.

Strategies of Prevention of Steal

a. Understanding the etiologies
b. Excluding and correction of arterial inflow disease
c. Careful evaluation the arteries of working extremity including the pressure and caliber of carotid, axillary, brachial, radial, and ulnar arteries, comparing the pressure and pulses with the contralateral side, especially if the pressure gradient is significant

between the proximal and distal part and between the left and right (usual > 15mmHg).

d. Detailed PE and ultrasound-based duplex images as cost-effective, non-invasive techniques which reveal the majority of vascular pathology.
e. Avoidance the usage of brachial artery as the inflow vessel in high-risk patients (see below)
f. The diameter of anastomosis of no more than 75% of inflow artery both in artery-to-vein or artery-to-graft (<7mm is usually mentioned); besides that some authors reported the use of non-smooth anastomosis (90 or 180 degrees) [10]
g. The use of tapered graft if the autogenous vessel is not available.
h. High-risk factors of steal including DM, female, brachial access, multiple
i. operations on the same limb, age over 60 year-old, DBI<0.45 (or 0.6), and intra-operative AV access flow over 2000 ml/min. Arterial atherosclerosis also contributes the risk of ischemia [3, 6, 39, 45].
j. Prevention is better than cure.

The Summary of Procedures to Deal with the Access Steal

- Banding
- Banding between dialysis puncture sites
- Minimally Invasive Limited Ligation Endoluminal-assisted Revision (MILLER) banding
- Access ligation
- Correction of the inflow lesion
- Transcatheter collateral veins coil embolization
- Ligation of the perforating vein
- Revision Using Distal Inflow (RUDI)
- Proximalization of arterial inflow (PAI)
- Distal Revascularization with Interval Ligation (DRIL)
- Ulnar artery dilatation

CONCLUSION

To date, the DRIL has been the most successful and widely accepted procedure for treatment of dialysis access-associated steal syndrome, but it does not mean that any type of DASS should be treated with the revascularization or the DRIL procedure. Actually DRIL, RUDI, PAI, or axillary loop procedures all are shared similar physical principles. We should be concerned about the vascular conditions such as proximal artery, distal artery, collateral circulations, and the venous resistance, and make the differential diagnosis for the true ischemia, neuropathy, and the IMN, and perform detailed physical examinations including non-invasive and invasive procedures to find the etiology of DASS and then we can treat the patients with DASS successfully.

REFERENCES

[1] Papasavas PK, Reifsnyder T, Birdas TJ, Caushaj PF, Leers S. Prediction of arteriovenous access steal syndrome utilizing digital pressure measurements. *Vasc Endovascular Surg* 2003; 37:179-84.

[2] Rocha A, Silva F, Queiros J, Malheiro J, Cabrita A. Predictors of steal syndrome in hemodialysis patients. *Hemodialysis International* 2012; Apr 17. [Epub ahead of print]

[3] Zamani P, Kaufman J, Kinlay S. Ischemic steal syndrome following arm arteriovenous fistula for hemodialysis. *Vasc Med* 2009; 14: 371-6.

[4] Ariya SK, Tanigawa N, Kojima H, Komemushi A, Shomura Y, Hiraishi T.. Transcatheter coil embolization for steal syndrome in patients with hemodialysis access. *Acta Radiol* 2009; 1:28-33.

[5] Tynan-Cuisinier GS, Berman SS. Strategies for predicting and treating access induced ischemic steal syndrome. *Eur J Vasc Endovasc Surg* 2006; 32: 309-15.

[6] Wixon CL, Hughes JD, Mills JL. Understanding strategies for the treatment of ischemic steal syndrome after hemodialysis access. *J Am Coll Surg* 2000;191: 301-10.

[7] Berman SS, Gentile AT, Glickman MH. Distal revascularization-interval ligation for limb salvage and maintenance of dialysis access in ischemic steal syndrome. *J Vasc Surg* 1997; 26: 393–402, discussion 402–4.

[8] Morsy AH, Kulbaski M, Chen C. Incidence and characteristics of patients with ischemia after hemodialysis access procedure. *J Surg Res* 1998; 74: 8–10.

[9] DeCaprio JD, Valentine RJ, Kakish. Steal syndrome complicating hemodialysis access. *Cardiovasc Res* 1997; 5: 648–53.

[10] Tordoir J H M, Dammers R, van der Sande FM. Upper extremity ischemia and hemodialysis vascular access. *Eur J Vasc Endovasc Surg* 2004; 27: 1–5.

[11] Duncan H, Ferguson L, Faris I. Incidence of the radial steal syndrome in patients with Brescia fistula for hemodialysis: its clinical significance. *J Vasc Surg* 1986; 4: 144–76.

[12] Furchgott RF, Zawadzki JV. The obligatory role of endothelial cells in relaxation of arterial smooth muscle by acetylcholine. *Nature* 1980; 288: 373-6.

[13] Anderson CB, Etheredge EE, Harter HR, Codd JE, Graff RJ, Newton WT. Blood flow measurements in arteriovenous dialysis fistulas. *Surgery* 1977; 81: 459–61.

[14] Schanzer H, Skladany M, Haimov M. Treatment of angioaccess-induced ischemia by revascularization. *J Vasc Surg* 1992; 16: 861–6.

[15] Haimov M, Schanzer H, Skladani M. Pathogenesis and management of upper-extremity ischemia following angioaccess surgery. *Blood Purif* 1996; 14: 350–4.

[16] Katz S, Kohl RD. The treatment of hand ischemia by arterial ligation and upper extremity bypass after angioaccess surgery. *J Am Coll Surg* 1996; 183: 239–42.

[17] Stierli P, Blumberg A, Pfister J, Zehnder C. Surgical treatment of steal syndrome induced by arteriovenous grafts for hemodialysis. *J Cardiovasc Surg* 1998; 39: 441–3.

[18] Knox RC, Berman SS, Hughes JD, Gentile AT, Mills JL. Distal revascularization - interval ligation: a durable and effective treatment for ischemic steal syndrome after hemodialysis access. *J Vasc Surg* 2002; 36: 250–5.

[19] Goff CD, Sato DT, Bloch PH, et al. Steal syndrome complicating hemodialysis access procedures: can it be predicted. *Ann Vasc Surg* 2000; 14: 138–44.

[20] Lazarides MK, Staramos DN, Kopadis G, Maltezos C, Tzilalis VD, Georgiadis GS. Onset of arterial 'steal' following proximal angioaccess: immediate and delayed types. *Nephrol Dial Transplant* 2003; 18: 2387–90.

[21] Wilbourn AJ, Furlan AJ, Hulley W, et al. Ischemic monomelic neuropathy. *Neurology* 1983; 33: 447-51.

[22] Bolton CF, Driedger AA, Lindsay RM. Ischemic neuropathy in uremic patients caused by bovine arteriovenous shunts. *J Neurol Neurosurg Psychiatry* 1979; 42: 810-4.

[23] Hye RJ, Wolf YG. Ischemic monomelic neuropathy: an under-recognized complication of hemodialysis access. *Ann Vasc Surg* 1994; 8: 578-82.

[24] Shemesh D, Goldin I, Olsha O. Banding between dialysis puncture sites to treat severe ischemic steal syndrome in low flow autogenous arteriovenous access. *J Vasc Surg* 2010; 52: 495-8.

[25] Zanow J, Petzold K, Petzold M, Krueger U, Scholz H. Flow reduction in high-flow arteriovenous access using intraoperative flow monitoring. *J Vasc Surg* 2006; 44: 1273–8.

[26] Shemesh D, Olsha O, Mabjeesh NJ, Abramowitz HB. Dialysis access induced limb ischemia corrected using quantitative duplex ultrasound. *Pediatr Nephrol* 2001; 16: 409-11.

[27] National Kidney Foundation-Dialysis Outcome Quality Innitiative. Clinical practice guidelines for vascular access: update 2000. *Am J Kidney Dis* 2001; 37(suppl 1): S137-81.

[28] Plumb TJ, Lynch TG, Adelson AB. Treatment of steal syndrome in a distal radiocephalic arteriovenous fistula using intravascular coil embolization. *J Vasc Surg* 2008; 47: 457-9.

[29] Miller GA, Goel N, Friedman A, Khariton A, Jotwani MC. The MILLER banding procedure is an effective method for treating dialysis-associated steal syndrome. *Kidney Int* 2009;77: 359–66.

[30] Jennings WC, Brown RE, Ruiz C, Tulsa, Okla. Primary arteriovenous fistula inflow proximalization for patients at high risk for dialysis access-associated ischemic steal syndrome. *J Vasc Surg* 2011; 54: 554-8.

[31] Schanzer H, Skladany M, Knight R, et al. Ischemia following angioaccess surgery. In: Veigh F, ed. *Current Critical Problems in Vascular Surgery,* vol. 7. St. Louis, Quality Medical Publishing; 1996: 484-6.

[32] Korzets A, Kantarovsky A, Lehmann J, Sachs D, Gershkovitz R, Hasdan G. The ``DRIL" Procedure - A neglected way to treat the "Steal" syndrome of the hemodialysed patient. *IMAJ* 2003; 5: 782-5.

[33] Wixon CL, Mills JL, Berman SS. Distal revascularization—interval ligation for maintenance of dialysis access and restoration of distal perfusion in ischemic steal syndrome. *Semin Vasc Surg* 2000; 13: 77–82.

[34] Huber TS, Brown MP, Seeger JM, Lee WA. Midterm outcome after the distal revascularization and interval ligation (DRIL) procedure. *J Vasc Surg* 2008; 48: 926-33.

[35] Scotts. Berman SS. Understanding Steal Syndrome: Causes and prevention strategies to prevent the development of significant VASS. *Endovascular Today* 2009; 71: 70-2.

[36] Reifsnyder T, Arnaoutakis GJ. Arterial pressure gradient of upper extremity arteriovenous access steal syndrome: treatment implications. *Vascular and Endovascular Surgery;* 44: 650-3.

[37] Minion DJ, Moore E, Endean E. Revision using distal inflow: a novel approach to dialysis-associated steal syndrome. *Ann Vasc Surg* 2005; 19: 625-8.

[38] Andrade JL, Paschoa AF, van Bellen B. Bridge graft to a small distal artery after fistula ligation for angioaccess-induced ischemia: report of two cases. *J Vasc Access* 2004; 5: 33-5.

[39] Callaghan CJ, Mallik M, Sivaprakasam R, Iype S, Gavin J. Treatment of dialysis access-associated steal syndrome with the "revision using distal inflow" technique. *J Vasc Access* 2011; 12: 52-6.

[40] Gradman WS, Pozrikidis C. Analysis of options for mitigating hemodialysis access-related ischemic steal phenomena. *Ann Vasc Surg* 2004; 18: 59-65.

[41] Fillinger MF, Reiwitz ER, Schwartz RA. Graft geometry and venous intimal-medial hyperplasia in arteriovenous loop grafts. *J Vasc Surg* 1990; 11: 556-66.

[42] Zanow J, Kruger U, Scholz H. Proximalization of the arterial inflow: a new technique to treat access-related ischemia. *J Vasc Surg* 2006; 43: 1216–1221; discussion 1221.

[43] Jendrisak MD, Anderson CB. Vascular access in patients with arterial insufficiency. *Ann Surg* 1990; 212: 187-93.

[44] Dyck PJ, Karnes JL, OBrien P. The spatial distribution of fiber loss in diabetic polyneuropathy suggests ischemia. *Ann Neurol* 1986; 19: 440-9.

[45] Mwipatayi BP, Bowles T, Balakrishnan S, Callaghan J, Sieunarine K. Ischemic steal syndrome: A case series and review of current management. *Curr Surg* 2006; 63: 130-5.

In: Fistuals and Fissures
Editors: Dmitri Pavlovich and Sergei Ivanovich ISBN: 978-1-62618-068-0

Chapter 7

ANAL FISSURE

Joseph Lysy[*] and Ariella Bar-Gil Shitrit
Digestive Disease Institute, Shaare Zedek Medical Center
Affiliated to the Hebrew University Medical school, Jerusalem, Israel

ABSTRACT

Anal fissures are common proctologic problems, associated with significant morbidity. Careful clinical evaluation to distinguish primary from secondary anal fissure is mandatory.

Anal fissure may have underlying pathology such as Crohn's disease, the prevalence of this disease significantly increased in the western countries in the last decades. Cancer and syphilis are other possible underlying diseases.

It is also important to distinguish anal fissures with high anal tone from those with normal anal tone.

Low anal tone and secondary soiling can provoke anoderm laceration which can mimic anal fissure, in this case chemical or surgical sphincterotomy may aggravate the anoderm injury.

Surgical and chemical sphincterotomy are both accepted treatments for chronic anal fissure. No single treatment is best choice for all patients. Both treatments modalities are much improved in the last decades. We use now combination and sequential pharmacotherapy e.g. calcium blockers, nitric oxide donors and botulinum toxin on one hand. On the other hand new surgical approaches providing lower risk of incontinence compared to the past and high healing rate. Impairment of anal sphincter by surgical procedure may cause immediate and delayed incontinence. On the other hand pharmacotherapy is much slower treatment modality with higher recurrence rate and increased risk for fissure infection and fistula formation.

Therefore treatment for anal fissure has to be tailored to the individual patients, taking in consideration the level of pain, and the potential individual risk for incontinence.

[*] Corresponding author Email: lysyj@szmc.org.il.

Introduction

Anorectal complaints are very common and are mostly caused by benign anorectal disorders. One of the most common causes of anorectal pain is anal fissure. It was first recognized as a disease in 1934 [1] and currently affects 10% of patients attending proctology clinics [2]. Fissures occur in all age groups, most commonly in 30- to 50-year-olds. Men and women have equal prevalence. Contrary to traditional teaching, a precipitating history of constipation is found only in small percentage of patients (approximately 20%) [3]. The majority of anal fissures are idiopathic. Possible causes include traumatic injury to the anal canal (such as with passage of a hard stool or severe diarrhea), infection, and hypertension of the anal sphincter.

Definition

An anal fissure is a cut or split in the epithelial lining of the anal canal distal to the dentate line. A chronic anal fissure is categorized when the fissure fails to heal within 6-8 wk. Chronic fissures develop ulceration and heaped-up edges with exposure of the internal anal sphincter fiber at the base of the ulcer. There is often an associated external skin tag and/or an internal hypertrophied anal papilla. The vast majority of anal fissures occur in the posterior midline, while 10% to 15% occur in the anterior midline [4] where it is more common in women than in men, and less than 1% of fissures occur in lateral positions.

If an anal fissure develops in atypical locations, one must consider other diseases. Crohn`s disease is the most common cause of anal fissures associated with atypical locations, although other inflammatory bowel diseases, syphilis, tuberculosis, leukemia, cancer and human immunodeficiency virus (HIV) are also known causes [5, 6].

Pathogenesis

The pathogenesis involves a cycle of repeated trauma and injury. Although the etiology of this condition is uncertain, the main hypothesis is that the posterior midline area may have decreased blood flow due to the configuration of the vessels of the anus [7]. Also, spasm of the internal anal sphincter may cause further reduction in blood flow to the posterior anal canal. Trauma from such factors as hard stools can aggravate the condition, and then eventually cause fissures. Recent research has shown the blood flow to the posterior midline of the anus to be potentially deficient, being supplied by end arteries (mean arteriolar blood pressure 85mmHg) which pass through the internal anal sphincter before reaching the posterior commissure [8]. As the maximum resting anal pressure (MRAP) is usually greater than 90mmHg in patients with fissures [9] such hypertonia will compress these end arteries and cause ischemia of the posterior commissure. Such a reduction in the posterior anodermal blood flow has been confirmed using laser Doppler flowmetry [10]. Further evidence that the hypertonia is not secondary to pain arises from the demonstration that it is not relieved by the use of topical anesthetics [11]. Once a tear occur, the internal anal sphincter muscle, which is exposed beneath the tear, goes into spasm and increased contraction, pulling the edges of the fissure apart, and impairing wound healing and leading to further tearing of the anal mucosa with subsequent passage of bowel movements. In addition, ischemia can contribute to the development of chronic anal fissure. Patients with chronic anal fissures also appear to have increased resting pressure in the anus per anal manometry [12, 13].

CLINICAL PRESENTATION AND DIAGNOSIS

Anal fissures can be diagnosed through history and physical examination. Patients present with the main complaint of a tearing pain, especially with and following defecation. It can be accompanied by bright red blood, which is usually limited to the surface of the stool or as a stain on the toilet paper. Patients may report avoidance of a bowel movement secondary to pain. The pain appears out of proportion to the size and seriousness of the lesion, and the patient can appear very reluctant to undergo examination. Other less common symptoms include pruritus and mucous discharge [14, 15]. Physical examination of the anal canal can be difficult secondary to the patient's pain. The pain caused by a deep chronic fissure is even more excruciating than that associated with a sore tooth. It can last for several hours, thus turning the patient into a living wreck with bloodshot eyes – the patient is unable to sleep a wink. The patient shudders every time he thinks about his next bowel movements, and therefore he makes an effort to delay defecation for 2-3 days. As a result, constipation gets increasingly prolonged and the patient`s sufferings intensify.

The physical examination is classic in the presence of a fissure. Sphincter tone is markedly increased, and digital examination produces extreme pain. Visual inspection of the lower anal canal for a fissure (most commonly located in the posterior midline) can be done by spreading the patient's buttocks and gently averting the anal verge. Once a fissure has become chronic, it is more difficult to obtain complete resolution. A sentinel tag or "pile" is frequently observed protruding from the anus. The proximal end of the fissure may contain granulation tissue that is often confused with an anal polyp. The area around the fissure becomes sclerotic and appears white. The sphincter musculature can frequently be visualized at the base of the fissure

Digital examination of the anal canal and anoscopy may be attempted, and pretreatment with lidocaine ointment may facilitate the examination. If digital examination or anoscopy cannot be performed, but a fissure can be observed by inspection, these procedures can be performed following initial treatment when the patient is in less pain. However, if the diagnosis cannot be established it may be necessary to administer conscious sedation (e.g., midazolam) or possibly regional or general anesthesia to obtain the examination.

TREATMENT: GENERAL CONSIDERATIONS

Healing rate for chronic anal fissures left untreated or treated conservatively with stool softeners range from 8% to 51%. Surgery, typically lateral internal sphincterotomy, is still considered the gold standard in the treatment of chronic anal fissure, but it carries a risk of incontinence to stool or flatus. This reported risk ranges from 3% to 16% [16] and remains the biggest long-term fear of patients and physicians. Therefore usually we begin treatment with the least invasive modality despite knowing that the surgical option had the highest chance of resolving the fissure.

NON SURGICAL TREATMENT FOR ANAL FISSURE

Behavioral Treatment

Less than 50% of chronic anal fissure are associated with constipation [17]. Other patients develop obstructed defecation type constipation symptoms (dyssynergic defecation) secondary to the pain during defecation: they contract the anal sphincters instead of relaxation. Patients are encouraged and showed how to relax the pelvic floor muscles during defecation. Those patients who will continue to suffer from obstructed defecation even after fissure healing will need biofeedback treatment. By this method patients are trained to relax the pelvic floor striated muscle during defecation, and to increase abdominal pressure effectively. Other patient defers bowel evacuation because of the pain. It is important for patients to be in the habit of going immediately to the bathroom for defecation when they want to have a bowel movement. The continuous holding of stools contributes to the vicious cycle of constipation by inhibiting neuromuscular reflex and decreasing sensation. Regular exercise such as walking eases defecation by facilitating colonic motility. High fiber diet and increased water intake should be encouraged. If these measures are not sufficient, bulk-forming laxatives are generally considered as a first-line drug, methylcellulose, and psyllium are examples of these agents. Hyperosmolar laxatives such as lactulose, and polyethylene glycol are second-line drugs. These drugs are not absorbed in the intestine and maintain high osmosis in the colon. Thus, defecation occurs in a soft form due to a lack of absorption of water into the body. Use of warm sitz baths may reduce pain and spasm. Local anesthetics can cause contact dermatitis and should not be used for long periods. These measures are sufficient for few patients these include those with a short history and in whom the fissure appears to be simple, superficial split without tag or papilla.

Pharmacological Treatment

The aim of pharmacological treatment for chronic anal fissure is to decrease the pressure in the anal canal and hence increase the blood flow with subsequent tissue healing. (Reversible chemical sphincterotomy). Topical nitrates, topical calcium channel blockers and botulinum toxin are the most widely used medications. Other options involves alpha – adrenoreceptor antagonists, beta- adrenoreceptor agonists and muscarinic agonists. Newer Pharmacological agents being tested include Gonayautoxin, a paralytic neurotoxin derived from shellfish [18]. The authors used topical hysdrocolloyds (Hydrogel) which is also available as a paste. Hydrocolloyds are used in practice for acute and chronic wounds such as diabetic foot ulcers [19].

Hydrocolloids are said to aid the healing by creating a moist environment and, through an intensification of the autolysis process. We used them as an adjuvant to muscle relaxants to promote wound healing.

Topical Nitrates

Nitric oxide is one of the most important inhibitory neurotransmitters involved in internal anal sphincter activity. As a nitric oxide donor, nitroglycerin (glyceryl trinitrate) ointment has become in many clinical contexts the first-line therapy for chronic anal fissure. The most common adverse reaction correlated with topical nitrates therapy is transitory headache occurring in an average of 25% of the patients, usually manageable in our experience by informing the patients regarding this side effect. Dose reduction (Very thin ointment layer) with gradual dose increase and, mild analgesics as needed [20, 21].

Glyceril trinitrate (GTN) has been tested mainly in two formulations: 0.2% and 0.4%. A study investigating the effect of GTN ointment concentrations on healing rates demonstrated a better healing rate with increasing concentrations (40.4% for 0.2% vs. 54.1% for 0.4%). Endoanal application of nitroglycerin ointment significantly reduces the frequency of headaches compared with perianal administration. The majority of the patients healed within 2 months. Once healing was achieved, recurrence does occur at a rate up to 50% [22, 23]. Isosorbide dinitrate, available commercially in the form of spray for cardiac patients, was used to treat patients with chronic anal fissure with 83% short term success [24].

Calcium Blockers

Have been described as causing relaxation of the smooth muscle of the internal anal sphincter. Oral and topical nifedipine have been shown to lower mean resting anal pressure [25, 26]. Topical nifedipine reduced maximum resting pressure by 11% healed significantly more chronic fissures at 6 weeks (95% vesus 16%), and produced no side effects [27].

In several countries in Europe and Israel industrially manufactured Nifedipine ointment with a formulation of 0.2-0.4% is available. Diltiazem ointment was used in several studies. The concentration tested varied among the studis but the most common dose was 2%, obtaining a cure in 75% of the patients [28]. In general calcium blockers treat anal fissure with the benefit of a lower incidence of side effects than topical nitrates. Topical therapy with diltiazem is rarely associated with headache and only incidentally perianal itch was observed. However fewer trails were conducted with calcium blockers in comparison to GTN [29].

What is the optimal duration of therapy for GTM and calcium blockers? In most studies 6-8 weeks is the recommended duration. In clinical practice treatment duration has to be tailored individually. A complete fissure healing or a stable scar has to be seen before treatment can be stopped. If follow up visits in proctologic clinic is not feasible, I recommend continuing treatment 1 month after pain relief. Pain reduction or relief is usually achieved within 2-4 weeks but healing is not complete, and an unstable scar can be seen for further several weeks. It seems that calcium blockers can be used safely during pregnancy and breastfeeding [30, 31].

Botulinum, Toxin

Botulinum toxin (BT) prevents muscular contraction through inhibiting the release of acetylcholine from peripheral nerve cells into neuromuscular junctions and has been proposed as a treatment for chronic anal fissure since 1993. In randomized controlled trials the healing rate with BT ranged from 41%to 73.8% [32, 33]. Dosages used ranged from 15-50 units. The most common dosages were 20-25 units. The Optimal injection site was investigated in one study. Patients were treated with BT injections in the internal sphincter either on each side of the posterior midline or on each side of anterior midline and the authors concluded that injection of botulinum toxin in anterior midline resulted in improved lowering of resting anal pressure and produced an earlier healing result [34].

Low frequencies of adverse events were reported in clinical trials. The most frequent were temporary incontinence to flatus in approximately 10% of patients and to liquids and feces in approximately 5% of patients. Perianal hematoma, perianal thrombosis were described and rarely perianal abcess.

Botulinum toxin is contraindicated, in case of pregnancy and in case of neurological disease such as myasthenia, and amyotrophic lateral sclerosis. In 5 years follow up recurrence rate after botulinum toxin injection was 52.5% [35].

Combination Therapy

One study showed that at the end of 6 weeks combined Botulinum toxin injection and local application of Isosorbide Dinitrate spray (ID) in patients with chronic anal fissure who failed previous treatment with ID was more effective than BT alone, 66 % healing rate in the combination group versus 20% on BT alone ($p=0.025$) [36].

In another study Botulinum toxin injection alone was compared with a combination of Botulinum toxin and GTN ointment and showed a 47% healing rate with combination therapy compared to 27% with Botulinum toxin alone [37].

Comparative Study

In a prospective comparative study, overall cure rates between nitroglycerine ointment, diltiazem ointment, and botulinum toxin injection were similar at 54%, 53%, and 51%, respectively [38].

Surgical Management

When conservative measures fail, a surgical approach becomes necessary for the definitive management of the chronic anal fissure. Digital anal dilation of the anal canal for the treatment of anal fissure was first described in the 1860s and was reintroduced into anal fissure therapy in 1964. A high cure rate of 90% was reported [39].

Anal dilatation has been criticized for causing extensive damage to internal and external sphincters leading to incontinence (up to 51%). More recently anal dilatation with standardized methods such as pneumatic dilatation and anal dilators was introduced. These new techniques have achieved similar healing rates to sphincterotomy with a much lower incontinence rate compared to conventional finger anal dilatation. It is important to note that these studies only have small study Populations [40].

Cochrane Review of seven randomized controlled trials, comparing anal stretch with internal sphincterotomy significantly favored sphincterotomy over anal stretch for efficacy (OR ¼ 3.35; 95%CI ¼ 1.55–7.26) and incontinence to flatus or feces (OR ¼ 4.03; 95% CI ¼ 2.04–7.46) [41].

Because of the unacceptably high rates of anal incontinence following anal dilatation, most clinicians have abandoned this procedure. Another reason for preferring other surgical techniques was the high recurrence rate reported for anal dilatation 28.6%, which is much higher than that for sphincterotomy [42].

Since the description of the technique of lateral internal sphincterotomy (LIT) by Eisenhammer in the 1950 [43], the technique was revised and improved and it is considered now as the gold standard against which all treatments are compared. Lateral internal sphincterotomy , performed with an open or closed technique, involves an incision of an internal sphincter, distal to the dentate line, with the possible excision of the sentinel pile and the hypertrophied papillae.

Healing rates appear to be similar, in both techniques, with open techniques ranging from 93% to 95% and closed approaches ranging from 90% to 97%. There appears to be no difference in major incontinence rates, which range from 2% to 5%. Incontinence is the most serious complication of LIS. The majority are transient incontinence. Soiling usually mild with minor or no symptoms may occur in up to 10% of the patients. The recurrence rates ranges from 0-15% [44-46].

Other complications include bleeding, hematoma, abscess and fistula. Recent publication raised the possibility that fecal incontinence may present as a late complication of anal fissure surgery. Incontinence several years after LIS may be associated with other cofactors accumulating over time or, more likely, anal fissure surgery may accelerate the physiologic age-related weakening of the anal sphincter [47].

Studies comparing internal sphincterotomy with Botulinum toxin showed a higher healing rate and lower recurrence rate for spincterotomy. Studies comparing Glyceril trinitrate ointment to sphincterotomy showed similar results to Botulinum toxin studies [48].

Newer surgical therapies in chronic anal fissure management include anal fissurectomy or fissurotomy. Fissurectomy involves freshening of the anal fissure to allow healing, and this includes excision of the fissure edges, curetting or excision of the fissure base and possibly excision of sentinel skin tags and anal polyps. One study investigated the role of fissurectomy in combination with Botulinum toxin injection, and achieved a 93% healing rate within 16 wk and a temporary flatus incontinence rate of 7% that resolved within 6 wk [49].

Despite the promising results, the experience and follow up accumulated with these techniques is substantially lower compared to lateral sphicterotomy. More studies are required to confirm its safety and long term efficacy.

Flap anoplasty is also used in the treatment of chronic anal fissures. The procedures involve fashioning a local flap to cover the fissure defect. As flap procedures do not involve disruption of the internal anal sphincter the risk of incontinence is extremely low. Flap anoplasty particularly useful in patients with normal or low anal tone, in fissures secondary to obstetric trauma associated with internal sphincter disruption and recurrence after LIS. Flap anoplasty procedure have achieved good healing rates (81% to 98%), approaching those of lateral sphincterotomy, with minimal anal incontinence complications. Flap failure rates are however relatively high (5.9% to 11.8%) [50].

A recent report described a new technique of division of the internal sphincter, termed sphincterolysis. This technique involved the use of finger pressure over the internal sphincter fibers to produce a full thickness division of the fibers without breaching the anal mucosa. This study achieved healing rates of 96.5% with a 3.5% temporary incontinence rate that resolved in 97% of the affected patients within 1 month [51].

New Treatments

Gonyautoxin is a new pharmacological therapy to chronic anal fissure and the initial results are optimistic with 100% healing rate within 2 wk and no incontinence reported.

The mechanism of action of Gonyautoxin is the dose dependent reversible binding of the toxin to voltage-gated sodium channels on excitable cells, thereby producing a neuronal transmission blockage. This mechanism is similar to that for Botulinum toxin (BT) in that the effects are reversible and non-permanent and so this does not solve the fundamental problem of recurrence noted in BT injection. Long term follow-up is therefore needed to determine the recurrence rate [52].

Another innovative treatment method for chronic anal fissures is the usage of a posterior perineal support device to decrease recurrent trauma to the anus. The posterior perineal support device is aimed to help support and hold up the anococcygeal region just posterior to the posterior anal wall, hence providing pressure to the posterior aspect of the pelvic floor to counteract the pressure exerted by the feces. This confers two advantages, the first is the enhancement of the defecation reflex for effective defecation and decreased straining and the second is the reduction in tissue stretching and tension of the posterior perineum and levator ani muscles. The initial results show promise, with over 75% of patients expressing moderate or greater improvement in two or more symptoms associated with chronic anal fissures as well as a decrease in pain score from five to zero. This device may be used as an adjuvant to pharmacological therapies [53].

Conclusion

The diagnosis of chronic anal fissure is usually strait forward. However careful medical history and examination is essential in order not to miss secondary fissure, malignancy and infection. Thorough medical history and careful examination are important to assess the level of the pain, the impact on the quality of life and the extent of the fissure and fibrotic changes.

In the minority of cases, when the pain is intolerable and the chronic changes are prominent, patients will refer to surgery directly. However the risk of incontinence has to be discussed with the patient.

In the majority of the cases when the diagnosis of the anal fissure is established, chemical sphincterotomy should be considered for both ethical and economic reasons. The choice has to lie with the patient but the doctor`s responsibility is to inform him about the benefits and side effects of the available therapies for chronic anal fissure.

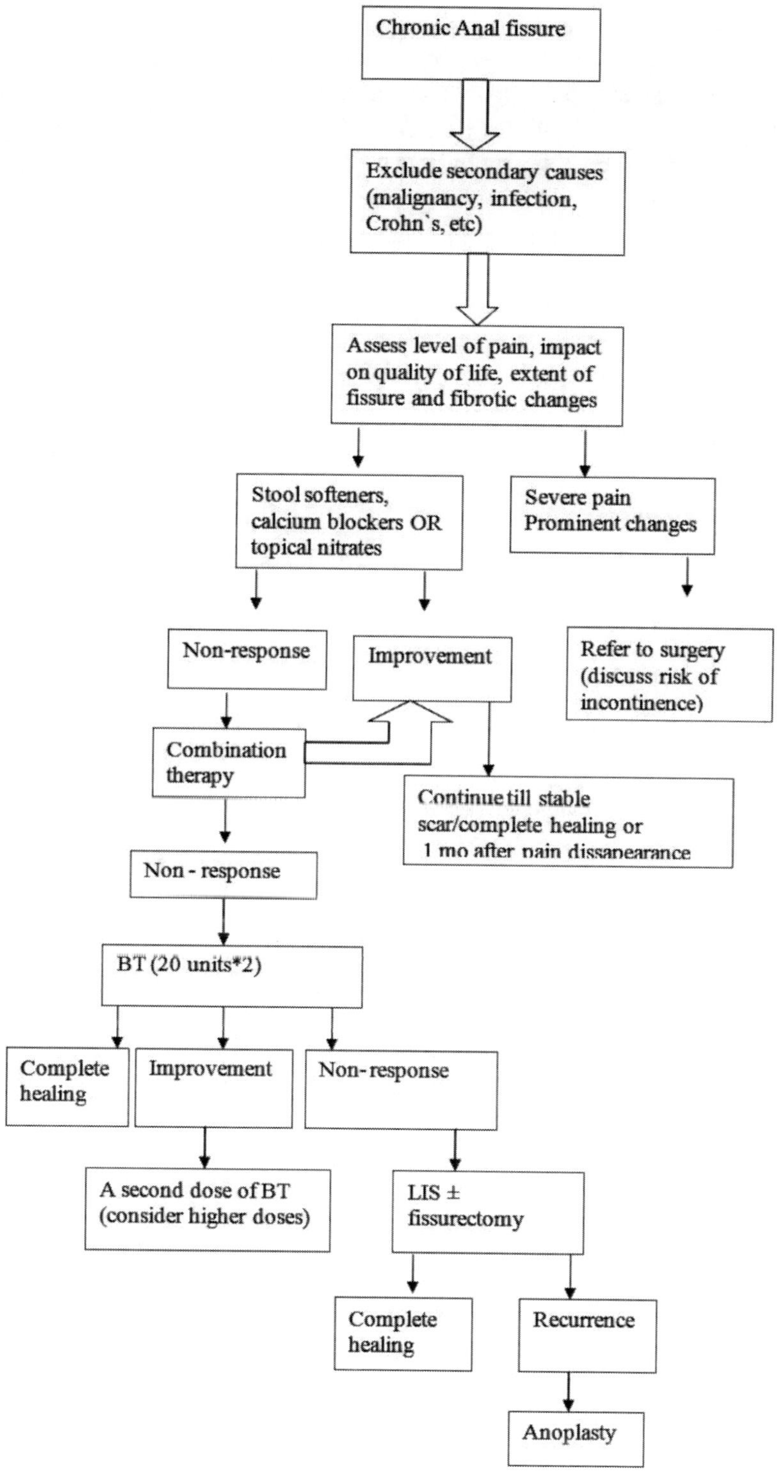

Figure 1. Algorithm for chronic anal fissure management.

In our experience most patients are willing to try less invasive modalities with the hope of avoiding surgery, with its risk of permanent disability.

All patients, regardless of specific treatment, have to be instructed on stool management to maintain soft stools at all times. Calcium blockers treat anal fissure with the benefit of a lower incidence of side effects than topical nitrates. However we can start with calcium blockers and switch to topical nitrates or vice versa in a case of side effects. Combination therapy in the case of non response is indicated. Treatment has to be continued until stable scar is seen or better when complete healing is achieved.

When regular visits by proctologist are not feasible, we suggest continuing treatment for 1 month after pain disappearance. Local application of Hydrogel on the fissure twice daily may accelerate fissure healing.

When the patient does not respond to nitrates, calcium blockers or combination of both drugs, then Botulinum toxin (BT) as a second line should be used. Injection of BT after local disinfection, 20 units each, bilaterally directly into the internal anal sphincter muscle (total dose 40 units). This step can be repeated a second time after 6 weeks if there were signs of improvement but not complete resolution. The optimal dose of BT has not been established. The dose may be related to anal sphincter mass anal tone and inflammation / fibrosis. Administration of higher doses of BT (50 or 80 units of Botox) could improve the results of chronic anal fissure therapy. Adding calcium blocker or local nitrate is advised but only one week after BT injection because minor incontinence is not unusual in the first week post BT injection.

Lateral internal sphincterotomy (LIS), either with or without fissurectomy and excision of sentinel skin tag, is the third line treatment. Anoplasty should be reserved for patients with normal or low anal tone and for those with recurrent fissure following LIS (Figure 1).

REFERENCES

[1] Lokhart Mummery JP. Diseases of the rectum and colon their surgical treatment. *Toronto MacMillan,* 1934.

[2] Pescatori M, Interisano A. Annual report of the Italian coloproctology units. *Tech. Coloproctol.,* 1995; 3:29-30.

[3] McCallion K, Gardiner K R. Progress in the understanding and treatment of chronic anal fissure. *Postgrad. Med. J.,* 2001; 77:753-758.

[4] Hananel N, Gordon PH. Re-examination of clinical manifestations and response to therapy of fissure-in-ano. *Dis. Colon. Rectum.,* 1997; 40:229-233.

[5] Fleshner P. Anal fissure in Crohn`s disease. *Semin. Colon. Rectal. Surg.,* 1997; 8:36-39.

[6] Saler ME, Gottesman L. Anal and rectal ulcer. In: Allen-Mersh TG, Gottesman I, editors. Anorectal Disease in AIDS. London: *Edward Arnold,* 1991:103 – 129.

[7] Smith LE. Anal fissures. Net J Med 1990;37 *Suppl.,* 1:S33-S36.

[8] Klosterhalfen B, Vogel P, Rixen H, et al. Topography of the inferior rectal artery: a possible cause of chronic, primary anal fissure. *Dis. Colon. Rectum.,* 1989; 32:43-52.

[9] Prohm P, Bonner C. Is manometry essential for surgery of chronic fissure-in-ano? *Dis. Colon. Rectum.,* 1995; 38:735-8.

[10] Schouten WR, Bricl JW, Auwerda JJ. Relationship between anal pressure and anodermal blood flow: The vascular pathogenesis of anal fissures. *Dis. Colon. Rectum.,* 1994; 37:664-9.

[11] Minguez M, Tomas-Ridocci M, Garcia A, et al. Pressure of the anal canal in patients with haemorrhoids or with anal fissure. Effect of the topical application of an anaesthetic gel. *Rev. Esp. Enform. Dig.*, 1992; 81:103-107.

[12] Gibbons CP, Read NW. Anal hypertonia in fissures: cause or effect? *Br. J. Surg.*, 1986; 73:443-445.

[13] Lin JK. Anal manometric studies in hemorrhoids and anal fissures. *Dis. Colon. Rectum.*, 1989; 32:839-842.

[14] Hancock BD: Anal fissures and fistulas. *BMJ*, 1992; 304:904.

[15] Mazier WP: Hemorrhoids, fissures, and pruritus ani. *Surg. Clin. North Am.*, 1994; 74:1277.

[16] Garcia-Aguilar J, Belmonte Montes C, Perez JJ, Jensen L Madoff RD, Wong WD. Incontinence after lateral internal sphincterotomy*: anatomic and functional evaluation Dis. Colon. Rectum.*, 1998; 41: 423–7.

[17] Hananel N, Gordon PH 1997 Re examination of clinical manifestation and response to therapy of fissure – in – *ano Dis. Colon. Rectum.*, 40;229-233.

[18] Garrido R, Lagos N, Lattes K et al. Gonyautoxin: new treatment for healing acute and chronic anal fissures. *Dis. Colon. Rectum.*, 2005; 48: 335–43.

[19] Edwards J, Stapley S (2010) Debridement of diabetic foot ulcers. *Cochrane Database Syst. Rev.*, Issue 1, Art. No.: CD003556.)

[20] Nelson R. Non surgical therapy for anal fissure. *Cochrane Database Syst. Rev.*, 2006:CD003431.

[21] Nelson RL, Thomas K, Morgan J, Jones A. Non surgical therapy for anal fissure. *Cochrane Database Syst. Rev.*, 2012; 2:CD003431.

[22] Scholefield JH, Bock JU, Marla B, Richter HJ, Athanasiadis S, Pröls M, Herold A. A dose finding study with 0.1%, 0.2%, and 0.4% glyceryl trinitrate ointment in patients with chronic anal fissures. Gut, 2003;52:264–269.

[23] Kennedy ML, Sowter S, Nguyen H, Lubowski DZ. Glyceryl trinitrate ointment for the treatment of chronic anal fissure: results of a placebo-controlled trial and long-term follow-up. Dis. Colon. Rectum., 1999; 42:1000–1006.

[24] Lysy J, Israelit-Yatzkan Y, Sestiery-Ittah M, *et al.* Treatment of chronic anal fissure with isosorbide dinitrate: long term results and dose determination. *Dis. Colon. Rectum.*, 1998; 41:1406–10.

[25] Chrysos E, Xynos E, Tzovaras G, et al. Effect of nifedipine on rectoanal motility. *Dis. Colon. Rectum.*, 1996;39(2):212–6.20.

[26] Carapeti EA, Kamm MA, Phillips RK. Topical diltiazem and bethanecol decrease anal sphincter pressure and heal anal fissures without side effects. *Dis. Colon. Rectum.*, 2000; 43(10):1359-62.

[27] Perrotti P, Bove A, Antropoli C, Molino D, Antropoli M, Balzano A *et al.* Topical nifedipine with lidocaine ointment *versus* active control for treatment of chronic anal fissure:results of a prospective, randomized, double-blind study. *Dis. Colon. Rectum.*, 2002; 45: 1468–1475.

[28] Steele SR, Madoff RD (2006) Systematic review: treatment of anal fissure. *Aliment. Pharmacol. Ther.*, 24:247–257.

[29] Perry WB, Dykes SL, Buie WD, Rafferty JF. Practice parameters for management of anal fissures (3rd revision). *Dis. Colon. Rectum.*, 2010; 53: 1110-1115).

[30] American Academy of Pediatrics Committee on Drugs: the transfer of drugs and other chemicals into human milk. *Pediatrics,* 1994; 93(1):137-50.

[31] Magee LA, Schick B, Donnenfeld AE, Sage SR. The safety of calcium channel blockers in human pregnancy: a prospective, multi – center cohort study. *Am. J. Obstet. Gynecol.,* 1996;174(3):823-8.

[32] Arroyo A, Pérez F, Serrano P, Candela F, Lacueva J, Calpena R. Surgical vs. chemical (botulinum toxin) sphinterotomy forchronic anal fissure: long term results of a prospective randomized clinical and manometric study. *Am. J. Surg.,* 2005; 189:429–434.

[33] Massoud BW, Mehrdad V, Baharak T, Alireza Z. Botulinum toxin injection versus internal anal sphincterotomy for the treatment of chronic anal fissure. *Ann. Saudi. Med.,* 2005; 25:140–142).

[34] Maria G, Brisinda G, Bentivoglio AR, Cassetta E, Gui D, Albanese A. Influence of botulinum toxin site of injections on healing rate in patients with chronic anal fissure. *Am. J. Surg.,* 2000; 179:46–50.

[35] Abd Elhady HM, Othman IH, Hablus MA, Ismail TA, AboryiaMH, Selim MF. Long term prospective randomised clinical and manometric comparison between surgical and chemical sphincterotomy for treatment of chronic anal fissure. *S. Afr. J. Surg.,* 2009; 47:112–114).

[36] Lysy J, Israelit-Yatzkan Y, Sestiery-Ittah M, Weksler-Zangen S, Keret D, Goldin E Topical nitrates potentiate the effect of botulinum toxin in the treatment of patients with refractory anal fissure. *Gut,* 2001; 48:221–22.

[37] Jones OM, Ramalingam T, Merrie A, Cunningham C, George BD, Mortensen NJ, Lindsey I. Randomized clinical trial of botulinum toxin plus glyceryl trinitrate vs. botulinum toxin alone for medically resistant chronic anal fissure: overall poor healing rates. *Dis. Colon. Rectum.,* 2006; 49: 1574-1580.

[38] Gil J, Luján J, Hernández Q, Gil E, Salom MG, Parrilla P. Screening for the effectiveness of conservative treatment inchronic anal fissure patients using anorectal manometry. *Int. J. Colorectal. Dis.,* 2010;25(5):649-654.

[39] Watts JM, Bennett RC, Goligher JC. Stretching of anal sphincters in treatment of fissure-in-ano. *BMJ,* 1964; 2(5405):342–343.

[40] Renzi A, Izzo D, Di Sarno G, et al. Clinical, manometric, and ultrasonographic results of pneumatic balloon dilatation vs. lateral internal sphincterotomy for chronic anal fissure: a prospective, randomized, controlled trial. *Dis. Colon. Rectum.,* 2008; 51(1):121–127.

[41] Nelson RL. Operative procedures for fissure in ano. *Cochrane Database Syst. Rev.,* 2010 ;(1):CD002199).

[42] Jensen SL, Lund F, Nielsen OV, Tange G. Lateral subcutaneous sphincterotomy versus anal dilatation in the treatment of fissure in ano in outpatients: a prospective randomised study. *Br. Med. J., (*Clin Res Ed) 1984; 289: 528-530.

[43] Eisenhammer S. The surgical correction of chronic internal anal (sphincteric) contracture. *S. Afr. Med. J.,* 1951;25(28): 486–489.

[44] Arroyo A, Pérez F, Serrano P, Candela F, Calpena R. Open versus closed lateral sphincterotomy performed as an outpatient procedure under local anesthesia for chronic anal fissure: prospective randomized study of clinical and manometric long term results. *J. Am. Coll. Surg.,* 2004; 199(3):361–367.

[45] Wiley M, Day P, Rieger N, Stephens J, Moore J. Open vs. closed lateral internal sphincterotomy for idiopathic fissure in-ano: a prospective, randomized, controlled trial. *Dis. Colon. Rectum.*, 2004; 47(6):847–852.

[46] Kortbeek JB, Langevin JM, Khoo RE, Heine JA. Chronic fissure-in-ano: a randomized study comparing open and subcutaneous lateral internal sphincterotomy. *Dis. Colon. Rectum.*, 1992; 35(9):835–83.

[47] Avi Levin, Matan J. Cohen, Victoria Mindrul , Joseph Lysy. An extra care has to be taken in considering LIS for high risk patients, such as elderly, multiparous women and patients with previous proctologic surgeries. Delayed fecal incontinence following surgery for anal fissure. *Int. J. Colorectal. Dis.*, 2011 26:1595–1599.

[48] Menteş BB, Irkörücü O, Akin M, Leventoğlu S, Tatlicioğlu E. Comparison of botulinum toxin injection and lateral internal sphincterotomy for the treatment of chronic anal fissure. *Dis. Colon. Rectum.*, 2003; 46: 232-237.

[49] Soll C, Dindo D, Hahnloser D. Combined fissurectomy and botulinum toxin injection. A new therapeutic approach for chronic anal fissures. *Gastroenterol Clin. Biol., 2008*; 32: 667-670.

[50] Singh M, Sharma A, Gardiner A, Duthie GS. Early results of a rotational flap to treat chronic anal fissures. *Int. J. Colorectal Dis.*, 2005; 20: 339-342.

[51] Gupta PJ. Closed anal sphincter manipulation technique for chronic anal fissure. *Rev. Gastroenterol. Mex.*, 2008; 73: 29-32.

[52] Garrido R, Lagos N, Lattes K et al. Gonyautoxin: new treatment for healing acute and chronic anal fissures. *Dis. Colon. Rectum.*, 2005; 48: 335–43.

[53] Tan KY, Seow-Choen F, Hai CH, Thye GK. Posterior perineal support as treatment for anal fissures--preliminary results with a new toilet seat device. *Tech. Coloproctol.*, 2009; 13: 11-15.

In: Fistuals and Fissures
Editors: Dmitri Pavlovich and Sergei Ivanovich
ISBN: 978-1-62618-068-0

Chapter 8

Advantage of Surgical Treatment for Intracranial Dural Arteriovenous Fistulas: Clinical Experience and Review of Literatures

Naoki Kato[1, 3*], Toshihide Tanaka[1], Yuzuru Hasegawa[1] and Toshiaki Abe[2]

[1]Department of Neurosurgery,
Jikei University School of Medicine Kashiwa Hospital,
Chiba, Japan
[2]Department of Neurosurgery,
Jikei University School of Medicine, Tokyo, Japan
[3]Department of Neurosurgery,
Charité Universitätsmedizin Berlin, Germany

Abstract

Overview: Dural arteriovenous fistulas (AVF) are relative infrequent neurovascular diseases. Since they have abnormal pathways between dural arteries and draining veins, venous infarction or intracerebral hemorrhage (ICH) can be caused by venous congestion. Pathophysiology and etiology are different between arteriovenous malformation (AVM) and AVF. Besides, pathogenesis of dural AVF yet remains unclear. They are usually treated with endovascular surgery. However, transarterial or transvenous embolization often fails to obliterate AVF completely due to cumbersome access and angiographically occult fistulas, which may result in recurrence. Therefore, direct surgery is also important modality for achieving complete therapeutic cure. Here we describe the advantages of direct surgery and review previous literatures including our clinical experience.

---

* Corresponding to:Naoki Kato, M.D., Ph.D.; Department of Neurosurgery; Jikei University School of Medicine Kashiwa Hospital; 163-1 Kashiwa-shita, Kashiwa, Chiba 277-8567, Japan; Tel: +81-3-3433-1111; Fax:+81-3-3459-6412 Ext. 3461; E-mail: nao-kth@jikei.ac.jp.

Role of Direct surgery for Intracranial AVF: Spinal AVFs can be favorably ligated with direct surgery. If intracranial, most of AVFs in the anterior cranial fossa are treated with craniotomy due to difficulty and risk of endovascular approach. On the other hands, direct surgeries for other locations are rarely reported, especially if main drainers were Sylvian vein or deep venous systems such as basal vein of Rosenthal. In these contexts, some cases underwent craniotomy following endovascular surgeries ended in fail. If the fistulas were successfully obliterated, the symptoms improved dramatically. Advantage of open surgery is considered that fistular points and microvessels on the dura can be cauterized and obliterated directly. Further surgical experience is demanded for adequate evidence to expand the validity of direct surgery for the intracranial AVFs.

Pial Fistula: Pial fistulas are rare vascular malformations. The structure of pial fistula is single channel between artery and venous system on the cortex without interventing abnormal vessels (e.g. nidus). As they can cause recurrence unless adequately occluded, potential existence of the pial fistula should be taken care. Conventional digital subtraction angiography (DSA) can hardly identify the pial fistulas, nevertheless, it is usually impossible to obliterate them via endovascular route. Therefore direct surgery plays a quite important role for detection and obliteration of pial fistulas.

Intraoperative Indocyanine Green (ICG) videoangiography for AVF: Currently intraoperative ICG videoangiography has become an indispensable tool for surgeries of several neurovascular lesions. It provides high resolution images of blood flow intraoperatively. For dural AVFs, ICG videoangiography can visualize not only the microvasculature but also residual pial fistulas.

Conclusion and Prospect: Complete detection and obliteration of fistular points, as well as, preservation of normal blood flow are recommended for the treatment of intracranial dural AVFs. We believe craniotomy is one of the most favorable treatments for these purposes. Additionally it enables us to obtain specimens of the dura containing fistula and microvasculature, which can develop the understanding about the pathophysiology of AVF. Finally the progress of intraoperative monitoring including ICG videoangiography will provide safe and accurate surgery and has a potential to study flow dynamics of dural AVF for appropriate therapeutic strategy. New generation of ICG videoangiography (FLOW800, Carl Zeiss) will be able to analyze flow dynamics of these vascular malformations.

A. Overview

Intracranial duralarteriovenous fistulas (AVF) are relative infrequent neurovascular diseases. Previously their incidence is reported as 10 to 15% of all intracranial arteriovenous malformations (AVM) [2]. Since they have abnormal pathways between dural arteries and draining veins, venous infarction or intracerebral hemorrhage (ICH) due to venous congestion can be induced as leading strokes [1, 23, 35]. Although they are similar to AVM, the pathology and mechanism are different. Besides, the cause of dural AVF is unclear yet. Some literatures occasionally reported that sinus or venous thrombosis was considered as one of causes [8, 25, 29, 35]. Infection, trauma and even operation might be the promoter of the AVFs [14, 15]. Despite the non-malignant pathogenesis, the prognosis of patients with AVF can be worsened progressively if not adequately treated [8].

Most popular grading scales of AVF were described by Cognard et al., Bordcn et al. and Lalwani et al. [3, 5, 22]. In each context, AVFs are classified according to venous drainage pattern which is correlated to patient's outcome [37]. Therefore the existence of tortuous or dilated vein is an important findings indicating venous congestion which should be treated.

Otherwise, following bleeding or venous infarction will affect the patient's prognosis for a long term period [1, 35].

They are usually treated with endovascular surgery, because of non-invasiveness and accessibility [24]. For instance, carotid cavernous fistulas are often treated by endovascular surgery and adequately occluded. However, for AVFs in other locatios, such as transverse sinus or convexity sinus, transarterial or transvenous embolization often fails to obliterate AVF completely resulting in recurrence [2, 13, 15, 38]. Therefore, direct surgery is also important modality for achieving complete therapeutic cure. Here we would like to describe the advantages of direct surgery and review previous literatures with our clinical experience. Recently we experienced two cases with intracranial dural AVF which was easy to access and successfully treated with radical surgical resection [18, 34]. Furthermore, we encountered a pial fistula adjacent to AVF in one of our cases [18]. Indocyanine green (ICG) videoangiography disclosed not only precise structure of the AVF but also an occult pial fistula intraoperatively. The entity of the pial fistulas with AVF is also rare and unique. In our experience, direct surgery is the most favorable maneuver for detection and adequate occlusion of angiographically occult fistula [18]. Direct surgery combined with intraoperative ICG videoangiography will be suggested to be safer and more accurate management of AVFs.

B. Role of Direct Surgery for Intracranial AVF

The role of direct surgery for the treatment of AVF has 2 patterns. One is direct occlusion of fistular points and the other role is exposure of vessels connecting to AVF for obtaining the access route for following endovascular surgery which could not be approached via only femoral cannulation [2, 36]. AVFs are found in both intracranial space and spinal lesion [6]. Spinal AVFs are the abnormal shunt between radicular arteries and medullary vein. The patients with spinal AVF suffer from myelopathy derived from venous congestion (e.g. Foix-Alajouanine syndrome). The ligation of draining vein is generally recommended and frequently performed [20, 28]. We can directly observe the vessels incorporated to the AVF [6]. In contrast, direct surgery for intracranial AVF is not so common, and published reports are not so many [32]. Exceptionally AVFs in the anterior cranial fossa are usually treated with direct surgery due to difficulty to access via endovascular route. The endovascular approach often fails to access the fistula points and even cause intraoperative complications such a bleeding caused by perforation, and so on [24].

Ultimate purpose of AVF treatment is to disconnect of all abnormal pathways between arterial feeders and draining veins [12]. Usually many arterial vasculatures are feeding fistula point (Figure 1a).

And ideal treatment is to occlude simply fistula point (Figure 1b). Arterial embolization is frequently performed, however, if some feeders were embolized incompletely, residual feeders will keep patency to the fistula point (Figure 1c). Moreover, caliber of residual feeders will increase again and even new fistulas could be induced, which leads to recurrence and progression of venous congestion (Figure 1d). On the other hand, obliteration of draining vein is performed at distant from the fistula point (Figure 1e), venous congestion could be worsened and might cause vessel collapse resulting in bleeding (Figure 1f).

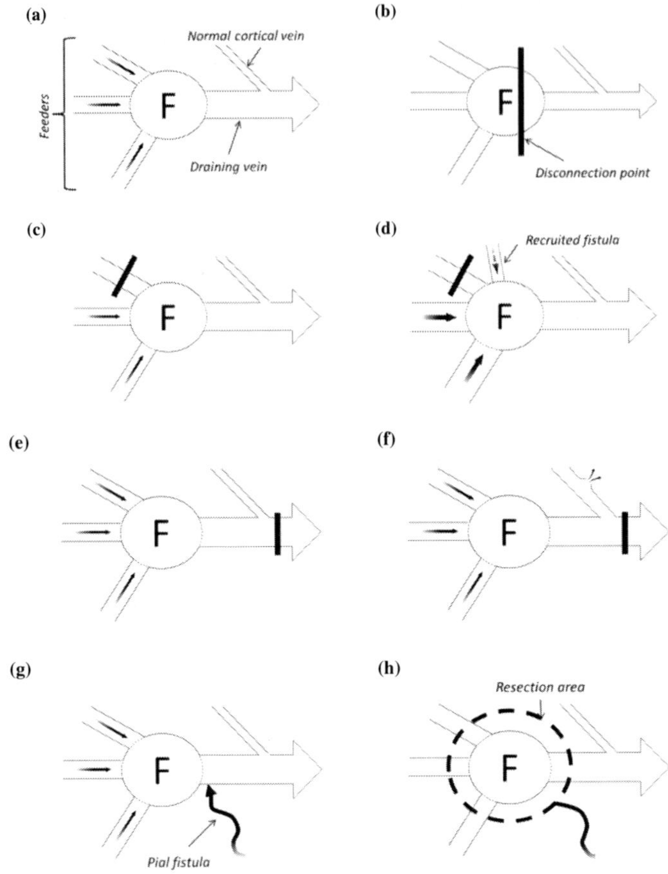

Figure 1 *Schema of AVF and each treatment*. Structure of AVF before treatment illustrating fistula point which is fed by 3 arterioles (a); "F" in the schema indicates the fistula point. The blood flow from the fistula point is drained into large caliber draining vein. Normal cortical vein is also connecting the draining vein. Theoretical concept of ideal ligation between feeding arteries and draining vein without interrupting normal venous flow (b). An example of partial arterial embolization and residual fistulas (c). Residual fistulas might have larger caliber than before and even a new recruited fistula can be induced after incomplete obliteration of AVF (d). Undesirable obstruction of AVF, i.e. distal migration of embolization material (e). Normal venous flow is disturbed and the cortical vein was dilated resulting venous congestion or collapse of the vessel (f). Special pattern of AVF indicating micro pial fistula between cortical artery and draining vein (g). Adequate resection of fistularpoint including the pial fistula can contribute the complete obstruction of abnormal pathways between arteries and draining vein without any interference of the normal venous flow (h).

Therefore distal migration of embolization glue has such a risk of intraoperative or postoperative complications [2, 13, 15, 38]. There is also special type of AVFs which are associated with pial fistulas (Figure 1g). It is difficult to identify or occlude them by endovascular approach [24]. Direct resection can achieve the complete obliteration of all fistula points (Figure 1h). Direct surgery is thought to be easier for obtaining accurate obliteration of AVF than endovascular surgery, if the access is possible.

We reviewed rare series of intracranial dural AVF which was surgically operated and similar to our cases. We conducted a literature search using the Pubmed site of the National Center for Biotechnology Information (http://www.ncbi.nlm.nih.gov/pubmed/).

Table 1. Features of previously reported cases with AVFs incorporated to Sylvian vein or basal vein of Rosenthal which was treated by surgical treatment

Study	Age, Sex	Location	Leading symptom	Draining vein	Preoperative EVS	Surgical approach	Postoperative course
Kadota et al. (1990)	52, M	Cavernous sinus	ICH	Rosenthal, Sylvian vein	+	Not mentioned	Improved
Ito et al. (1995)	49, M	Tentorium	Memory disturbance	ISS, Straight sinus, Rosenthal	+	OTA	Free
Bertalanffy et al. (2001)	57, M	Parasagittal convexity	ICH	Trolard, SSS	+	Parasagittal	Free
Kattner et al. (2002)	57, F	Tentorium SPS	Seizures	Leptomeningeal, Rosenthal	-	Anterior petrosal	Free
Nomura et al. (2002)	59, W	Middle fossa	SAH	Sylvian vein, Sphenobasal sinus	-	Subtemporal	Free
Gutiérrez-González et al. (2009)	73, M	Middle fossa	IVH	Rosenthal	-	Pterional	Not mentioned
Weil et al. (2011)	53, M	Tentorium	ICH	Rosenthal	+	Subtemporal	Improved
Tanaka et al. (2012)	61, M	Sphenoid ridge	Cerebral infarction	Rosenthal	-	Pterional	Free
Kato et al. (2012)	41, M	Convexity	ICH	Sylvian vein	-	Front-parietal craniotomy	Improved

SPS = superior petrosal sinus, SAH = subarachnoid hemorrhage, IVH = intraventricular hemorrhage, SSS = superior sagittal sinus, ISS = inferior sagittal sinus, Rosenthal = basal vein of Rosenthal, Trolard = anastomotic vein of Trolard, EVS = endovascular surgery, OTA = occipital transtentorial approach.

Our research was based on the following terms: “surgery”, “intracranial”, “convexity”, “anastomotic vein of Trolard”, “Sylvian vein”, “middle fossa” and “basal vein of Trolard”. All retrieved results were carefully reviewed for case descriptions that were included for subsequent analysis.

Reports in references of retrieved literatures were also viewed and included if they matched to the above criteria. Manuscripts which were not described in English were excluded from our investigation. Because of rare location and scarcely performed direct surgeries, the published cases were very limited, especially if main drainers were Sylvian vein or deep venous systems such as a basal vein of Rosenthal. In total, 9 cases, including our cases, were reviewed in the present manuscript (Table 1) [2, 9, 13, 15, 18, 19, 27, 34, 38].

Almost cases are man and initial symptoms are ICH or some neurological deficits due to venous congestion. And many cases were treated by endovascular surgery prior to the direct surgery. In these contexts, endovascular surgeries were usually performed via transarterial approach and resulting in recurrence. Then the craniotomy was decided in order to complete cure.

We guess all fistula points could not be obliterated via endovascular route, and residual feeders or even de novo arteriovenous connection could be induced as previously described. If the fistulas were successfully obliterated by the direct surgeries, the symptoms of published cases successfully improved. Further surgical experience is demanded for adequate evidence expanding validity of the direct surgery for the intracranial AVFs.

In our cases, standard craniotomies in a usual fashion could be applied for adequate exposure of fistula points (Figure 2) [18, 34]. For the convexity AVF, we could approach the fistula point more simply by craniotomy. In each surgical procedure, feeding arteries definitely transected such as extracranial arteries as the skin incision, and meningeal arteries as dural incision (Figure 3). Usually the fistula points need to be only ligated or coagulated.

However we tried to resect the fistula point for obtaining complete obliteration of AVF and specimen. This maneuver was not formidable method and avoided unnecessary occlusion of normal veins.

Besides, the direct surgery enables us to observe the color change of AVF vessels or apply intraoperative ICG videoangiography to confirm complete obliteration of abnormal draining veins. If necessary, the abnormal dura should be removed and replaced with artificial membrane (GORE-TEX sheet) which is considered to make enough distance between dural arteiroles and draining vein on the brain cortex [18].

It is now controversial whether the fistula need to be removed or obliteration of the fistula points alone is good enough [12]. In our experience, adequate craniotomy enables us to approach the AVF safely.

Beside, resection of all abnormal vasculature may be better for complete cure, even for particular cases with pial fistulas, and gives us a chance to examine the histopathological features of AVF. Histological findings indicated dilated vessels and lack of internal lamina of the wall, demonstrating fistula point.

As interesting findings particularly, hyalinized dura or multiple vasculature connecting to a venous vessel are also observed in the specimens as well. These histological findings suggest that chronic hypoxic condition derived from continuous venous hypertension might promote the angiogenesis and recruit microvasculature around the fistula points [18 34].

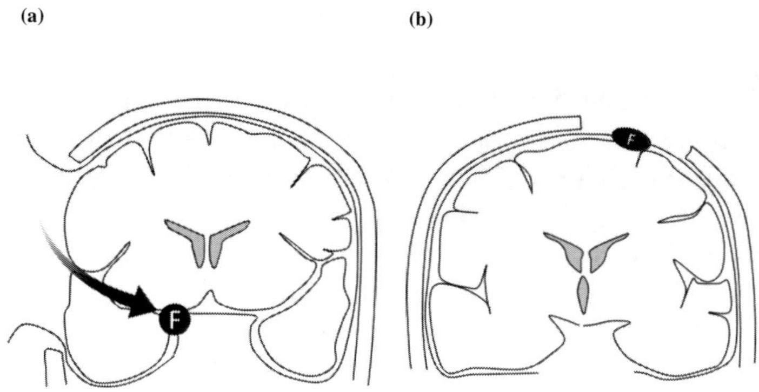

Figure 2. *Schema of approaches used for the treatment of intracranial AVF*. Image of coronal view showing an approach to the AVF locating near the lateral part of cavernous sinus (a); "F" in the schema indicates the fistula point. After the standard fronto-temporal craniotomy and opening of the dura mater, the Sylvian fissure was opened to approach the fistula point near sphenoid ridge. Schema of fronto-parietal craniotomy showing the fistula point which is located on convexity dura and can be safely exposed (b).

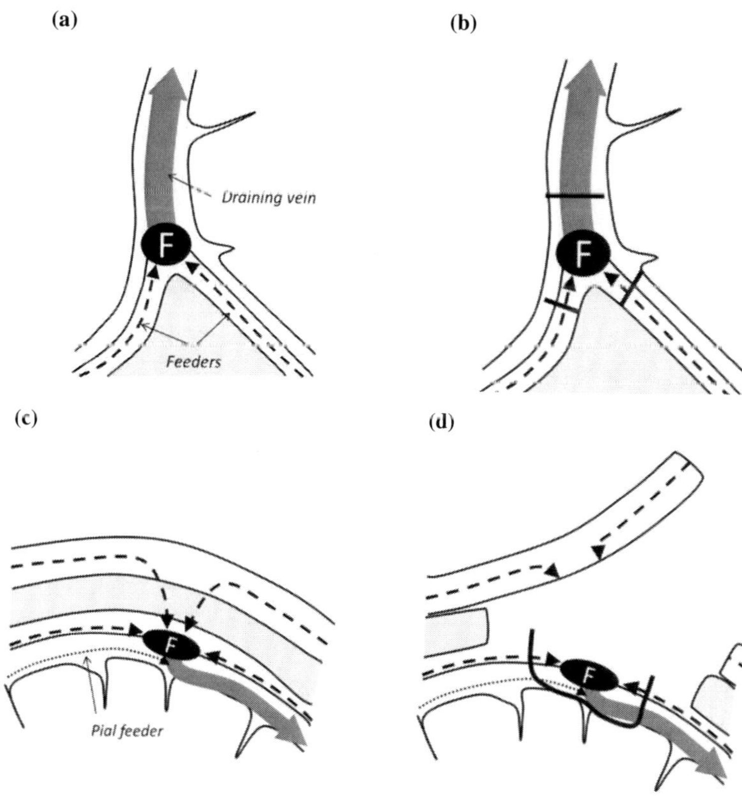

Figure 3. *Surgical strategy for AVF with and without pial fistula*. The structure of AVF fed by only dural arteries (a). This type can be obliterated by only dural incision and transection of the draining vein (b). Three black lines indicate the resection line. The structure of AVF fed by not only dural arteries but also a cortical artrery (pial fistula) (c). Feeders from scalp are occluded as skin incision and other feeders are transected with fistula point. This type should be resected with the pial fistula (d). "F" = fistula point.

C. Pial Fistulas

Pial fistulas are rare vascular malformations [12, 14, 31]. They are sometimes found with AVM, and have abnormal pathways between cortical arteries and draining veins. According to previous literatures, the incidence of the pial AVF is reported as 1.6% to 3.2% in the AVM [24, 31, 41]. The structure of pial fistula differs from AVM and is single channel between artery and venous system on the cortex without any interventing abnormal vessels (e.g. nidus) [16]. Acquired pial fistula such as following venous thrombosis and irradiation are previously reported [29, 31]. Other causes of pial fistulas are known as Osler-Weber-Rendu syndrome, Klippel-Trenaunay-Weber disease, Ehlers-Danlos syndrome, Galen aneurysms and neurofibromatosis Type I [24]. Since inadequate occlusion of pial shunt might induce recurrence of the fistula, potential existence of the pial fistula should be taken care.

Intraoperative Doppler sonography is one of the favorable methods to detect the existence of pial fistulas [16]. If residual pial fistulas are remained, Doppler sonography shows residual arterial wave in the draining vein [16]. Recent alternative tool is ICG videoangiography. ICG videoangiography has been frequently used, which might make it easy to visualize pial fistulas unexpectedly, leading to recognition and understanding of its existence. Conventional digital subtraction angiography (DSA) can hardly identify the pial fistulas, nevertheless, it is usually impossible to obliterate them via transcatheter therapy [31].

The reported complication rate of endovascular surgery for pial AVFs was 18.75% and there were often incomplete obliteration [24]. Therefore direct surgical operation plays a quite important role for detection and obliteration of pial fistulas. More frequent use of ICG videoangiography will be expected to disclose the actual incidence of pial fistula with intracranial dural AVF.

D. Intraoperative ICG Videoangiography for AVF

Currently intraoperative ICG videoangiography has become an indispensable modality for surgeries of several neurovascular lesions [30, 39]. ICG is a fluorescence dye that has been used for evaluation of cardiocirculatory, liver function and ophthalmic angiography. After the approval of food and drug administration (FDA) in 1970s, this technique was widely and safely performed [6]. After injection of ICG to the body, most of ICG in blood vessel contact to globulins. Usual dose of ICG is 25 mg per an angiography (the recommended dose of ICG dye for videoangiography is 0.2 to 0.5 mg/kg, and the maximum daily dose should not exceed 5mg/kg) [30]. Then they stay intravascular space and become fluorescent material with absorption and emission peaks which are 805 and 835 nm [39]. ICG will appear in short seconds after intravenous injection, and go through the exposed vasculatures with marked illumination [20]. In the operative field, the illumination of ICG can be recorded by near-infrared camera which is now mounted to a neurosurgical microscope (e. g. OPMI Pentero microscope, Carl Zeiss, Germany) [11]. Almost administered ICG is discharged by liver and promptly cleared (a plasma half -life is 2~4 minutes). This character enables us to perform frequent ICG videoangiography in the same operation. Minimal required time between two ICG videoangiography is 10 minutes [10].

It provides high resolution images of blood flow in concerned areas intraoperatively. Woitzik et al. described the reliability for bypass patency of STA-MCA bypass [39]. For the aneurysmal surgeries, ICG videoangiography can disclose the rest perfusion or confirm complete clipping [30]. With this technique, patency of perforators near the neck of aneurysm can be also secured [30]. Intraoperative DSA is a useful modality for these procedures as well [24]. However, this technique is not always available in every institute, and catheter dislocation, thromboembolism or radiation exposure are not ignorable complications [11, 24]. And ICG videoangiography is cost effective and easy to handle compared to intraoperative DSA [39].

Some reports have proven the helpfulness of intraoperative ICG videoangiography for AVM surgeries [10, 33]. After the dural opening, we can assess the localization and the vessel features (feeders or draining veins) with ICG illumination. This is quite supportive for dissecting accurate plane between normal brain tissue and nidus [10]. The use of ICG videoangiograpy for spinal AVFs are also often reported [6, 20]. Conventional DSA is common technique for the detection of spinal AVF. However there are also rare cases with DSA occult spinal AVF [6, 20]. Even if the precise location of fistular point was not identified by preoperative conventional DSA, intraoperative ICG videoangiography can visualize detailed structure of spinal AVF directly [20]. If accurate ligation was performed, videoangiography confirms the disappearance of ICG filling inthe vein [6, 20]. Besides, it will help us to preserve the normal circulatory system (e.g. normal veins, perforators) [6, 30].

Other potential capacity of ICG videoangiography is described in recent years. ICG videoangiography can also visualize vascular structures beneath the hemorrhagic clots [21]. Even if the concerned structure is hided under subarachnoid clot, ICG videoangiography can disclose the buried vasculatures [21]. Depth of operative field is known as a common limit of ICG videoangiography [7]. Nishiyama et al. introduced the use of endoscopic ICG videoangiography for the deep seated vascular structures in aneurysmal surgery [26].

On the other hand, the use of ICG videoangiography for intracranial AVF has been seldom reported so far. The complication of the intraoperative ICG videoangiography for dural AVF may be rare [32]. And the rate of obliteration confirmed by intraoperative ICG videoangiography correlated to the findings of postoperative conventional DSA [32]. Generally, the ICG videoangiography was used after dural opening [32]. However, in our experience, ICG videoangiography visualized whole view of the structure and flow dynamics prior to dural incision. And it contributed to decide adequate dural incision. Moreover, ICG videoangiography could display not only the structure but also residual pial fistulas [18]. We believe it will be the favorable modality for treating intracranial dural AVF.

E. Conclusion and Prospect

Complete detection and obliteration of fistula points, as well as, preservation of normal blood flow are recommended for the treatment of intracranial dural AVFs. We believe direct surgery is one of the most effective treatments forthese purposes. We have to occlude fistula points with direct exposure aggressively as far as possible. Additionally it enables us to obtain specimens of fistula points which can advance the understanding about the pathophysiology of AVF. Finally the progress of intraoperative monitoring devices including ICG videoangiography will make the surgery much safer and has a potential to study flow dynamics of dural AVF.

Currently, a new tool of ICG videoangiography (FLOW800, Carl Zeiss) has become available for clinical use. Injected ICG passes rapidly into the arterial, capillary and venous structures. The arrival time of the illumination can distinguish high and low velocity of cerebral blood flow. It provides colored map indicating time interval between half peak and appearance of ICG in the operative field (e.g. the rapid appearance is colored red and slow is blue). This picture can be calculated in 2 minutes after injection of ICG. Then, indeed, we can observe the flow velocity of exposed area at a glance intraoperatively. On the pathological field, such an ischemic core or arteriovenous shunt, the colored map will change in accordance with cerebral blood flow. This will help us to detect the feeders of AVM, or recognize the direction of blood flow in the vessels [4, 17]. Another function of FLOW800 is calculating the intensity diagram of ICG in concerned areas (Figure 4). We can put the regions of interest (ROI) everywhere we want [4]. Then FLOW800 software products the diagram immediately and calculates parameters regarding flow dynamics [17].

The first attempt to analyze the intensity diagramof ICG was studied by Woitzik et al. [40]. They performed ICG videoangiography for patients with huge middle cerebral artery infarction and recorded the intensity curve. In their context, the diagram could display 3 different patterns according to ischemic core, penumbra and oligemia. This method helps the surgeons to determine the adequate location on which the tissue probe should be placed [40].

(a)

(b)

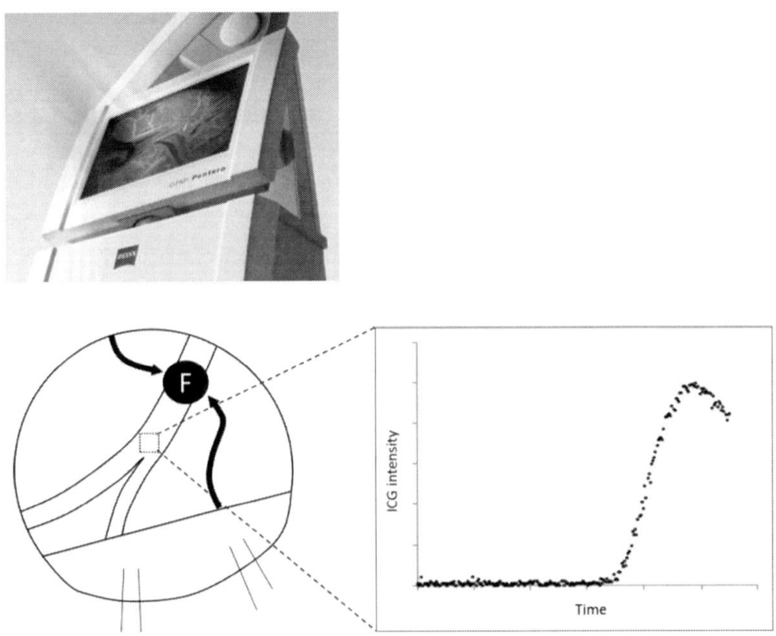

Figure 4. *Images of FLOW800 system.* An outward appearance of a microscope on which ICG videoangiography and FLOW800 system are mounted (Carl Zeiss GmbH, Germany)(a). Illustration demonstrating the concept of FLOW800 function (b). We can put ROIs on concerned vessels and measure the intensity of ICG. The diagram shows the intensity curve after appearance of ICG in the ROI.

Another known use of FLOW800 was described by Kamp et al. [17]. They applied the measurement for patients with aneurysms, AVMs and moyamoya diseases. And some parameters associated with cerebral blood flow were achieved. We hope that this tool will be able to analyze precise flow dynamics of AVFs. And for this purpose, further development of direct surgery is necessary to study the pathophysiology of AVFs.

ACKNOWLEDGMENT

The authors wish to thank Prof. P. Vajkoczy for his assistance with great suggestion.

REFERENCES

[1] Awad IA, Little JR, Akrawi WP, Ahl J. Intracranial arteriovenous malformations: factors predisposing to an agrressive neurological course. *J. Neurosurg.* 1990; 72, 839-850.

[2] Bertalanffy A, Dietrich W, Kitz K, Bavinzski G. Treatment of Dural Arteriovenous Fistulae (dAVF's) at the Superior Sagittal Sinus (SSS) Using Embolisation Combined with Micro- or Radiosurgery. *Minim. Invas. Neurosurg.* 2001; 44, 205-210.

[3] Borden JA, Wu JK, Shucart WA. A proposed classification for spinal and cranial dural arteriovenous fistulous malformations and implications for treatment. *J. Neurosurg.* 1995; 82, 166-179.

[4] Chen SF, Kato Y, Oda J, Kumar A, Watabe T, Imizu S, Oguri D, Sano H, Hirose Y. The application of intraoperative near-infrared indocyanine green videoangiography and analysis of fluorescence intensity in cerebrovascular surgery. *Surg. Neurol. Int.* 2011; 2:42.

[5] Cognard C, Gobin YP Pierot L, Bailly AL, Houdart E, Casasco A, Chiras J, Merland JJ. Cerebral dural arteriovenous fistulas: clinical and angiographic correlation with a revised classification of venous drainage. *Radiology*. 1995; 194(3), 671-680.

[6] Colby GP, Coon AL, Sciubba DM, Bydon A, Gailloud P, Tamargo RJ. Intraoperative indocyanine green angiography for obliteration of a spinal dural arteriovenous fistula. *J. Neurosurg. Spine.* 2009; 11, 705-709.

[7] Faber F, Thon N, Fest G, Rachinger W, Guckler R, Tonn JC, Schichor C. Enhanced analysis of intracerebral arteriovenous malformations by the intraoperative use of analytical indocyanine green videoangiography: technical note. *Acta. Neurochir.* 2011; 153, 2181-2187.

[8] Graeb DA, Dolman C. Radiological and pathological aspects of dural arteriovenous fistulas. *J. Neurosurg.* 2009; 151,1009-1012.

[9] Gutiérrez-González R, Boto GR, Rivero-Garvía M, Pérez-Zamarrón Á. Intraventricular haemorrhage caused by the rupture of a dural arteriovenous malformation of the middle cranial fossa. *Acta. Neurochir.* 1986; 64,962-967.

[10] Hänggi D, Etminan N, Steiger HJ. The Impact of Microscope-Integrated Intraoperative Near-Infrared Indocyanine Green Videoangiography on Surgery of Arteriovenous

Malformations and Dural Arteriovenous Fistulae. *Neurosurgery*. 2010; 67(4), 1094-1103.

[11] Hettige S, Walsh D. Indocyanine green video-angiography as an aid to surgical treatment of spinal dural arteriovenous fistulae. *Acta. Neurochir.* 2010; 152, 533-536.

[12] Hoh BL, Putman CM, Budzik RF, Ogilvy CS. Surgical and Endovascular Flow Disconnection of Intracranial Pial Single-channel Arteriovnous Fistulae. *Neurosrugery.* 2001; 49(6), 1351-1364.

[13] Ito M, Sonokawa T, Mishina H, Sato K. Reversible Dural Arteriovenous Malformation-induced Venous Ischemia As a Cause of Dementia: Treatment by Surgical Occlusion of Draining Dural Sinus: Case Report. *Neurosurgery*. 1995; 37, 1187-1192.

[14] Jimbo H, Ikeda Y, Izawa H, Otsuka K, Harada J. Mixed Pial-Dural Arteriovenous Malformation in the Anterior Cranial Fossa –Two Case Reports-. *Neurol. Med. Chir.* [Tokyo] 2010;50, 470-475.

[15] Kadota K, Asakura T, Kusumoto K, Kodama S, Okahara K, Miyanohara O, Kawasaki T, Kasamo S. Unusual Intra- and Extracranial Arteriovenous Communication. *Neurol. Med. Chir.* (Tokyo). 1990; 30, 753-758.

[16] Kakino S, Ogasawara K, Kubo Y, Ogawa A. Spontaneous pial single-channel arteriovenous fistulae with angiographically occult small feeding arteries: case report. *Surg. Neurol.* 2008;69, 187-191.

[17] Kamp MA, Slotty P, Turowski B, Etminan N, Steiger HJ, Hänggi D, Stummer W. Microsurgical integrated quantitative analysis of intra-operative indocyanine green fluorescence angiography for blood flow assessment: First experience in 30 patients. *Neurosurgery*. 2012;70(1 supple operative), 65-73.

[18] Kato N, Tanaka T, Suzuki Y, Sakamoto H, Arai T, Hasegawa Y, Abe T. Multistage Indocyanine Green Videoangiography for the Convexity Dural Arteriovenous Fistula with Angiographically Occult Pial Fistula. J Stroke Cerebrovasc Dis; doi:10.1016/j.jstrokecerebrovasdis.2012.05.008.

[19] Kattner KA, Roth TC, Giannotta SL. Cranial Base Approaches for the Surgical Treatment of Aggressive Posterior Fossa Dural Arteriovenous Fistulae with Leptomeningeal Drainage: Report of Four Technical Cases. *Neurosurgery*. 2002;50(5), 1156-1161.

[20] Killory BD, Nakaji P, Maughan PH, Wait SD, Spetzler RF. Evaluation of Angiographically Occult Dural Arteriovenous Fistulae with Surgical Microscope-Integrated Intraoperative Near-Infrared Indocyanine Green Angiography: Report of 3 Cases. *Neurosurgery*. 2011; 68(3), 781-787.

[21] Kuroda K, Kinouchi H, Kanemaru K, Wakai T, Senbokuya N, Horikoshi T. Indocyanine green videoangiography to detect aneurysm and related vascular structures buried in subarachnoid clots. *J. Neurosurg.* 2011; 114, 1054-1056.

[22] Lalwani AK, Dowd CF, Halbach VV. Grading venous restrictive disease in patients with dural arteriovenous fistulas of the transverse/sigmoid sinus. *J. Neurosurg.* 1993; 79, 11-15.

[23] Lasjaunias P, Chiu M, Brugge KT, Tolia A, Hurth M, Bernstein M. Neurological manifestations of intracranial dural arteriovenous malformations. *J. Neurosurg.* 1986; 64, 724-730.

[24] Lv X, Jiang C, Li Y, Yang X, Wu Z. Clinical Outcomes of Endovascular Treatment for Intracranial Pial Arteriovenous Fistulas. *World Neurosurg.* 2010; 73(4), 385-390.

[25] Mineta T, Fukuyama K, Koga H, Matsumoto S, Kishikawa T, Tabuchi K. Dural Arteriovenous Malformation Associated with Occlusion of the Superior Sagittal Sinus. *Neurol. Med. Chir.* (Tokyo)1991; 31, 41-44.

[26] Nishiyama Y, Kinouchi H, Senbokuya N, Kato T, Kanemaru K, Yoshioka H, Horikoshi T. Endoscopic indocyanine green video angiography in aneurysmal surgery: an innovative method for intraoperative assessment of blood flow in vasculature hidden from microscopic view. *J. Neurosurg*. 2012, 117(2), 302-308.

[27] Nomura S, Anegawa S, Nakagawa S, Tomokiyo M, Koga H, Hayashi T. Subarachnoid Hemorrhage Caused by Dural Arteriovenous Fistula of the Sphenobasal Sinus. *Neurol. Med. Chir.* (Tokyo) 2002, 42, 255-258.

[28] Ommaya AK, Chiro GD, Doppman J. Ligation of Arterial Supply in the Treatment of Spinal Cord Arteriovenous Malformations. *J. Neurosurg.* 1969; 30, 679-692.

[29] Phatouros CC, Halbach VV, Dowd CF, Lempert TE, Malek AM, Meyers PM, Higashida RT. Acquired Pial Arteriovenous Fistula Following Cerebral Vein Thrombosis. *Stroke*. 1999; 30, 2487-2490.

[30] Raabe A, Nakaji P, Beck J, Kim LJ, Hsu FPK, Kamerman JD, Seifert V, Spetzler RF. Prospective evaluation of surgical microscope-itegrated intraoperative near-infrared indocyanine green videoangiography during aneurysm surgery. *J. Neurosurg.* 2005; 103, 982-989.

[31] Saito A, Sugawara T, Mikawa S, Akamatsu Y, Saito H, Seki H. A case of multiple pial arteriovenous fistulas asscioated with dural arteriovenous fistula: Casse report. *J. Neurosurg.* 2008; 109, 1103-1107.

[32] Schuette AJ, Cawley CM, Barrow DL. Indocyanine Green Angiography in the Management of Dural Arteriovenous Fistulae. *Neursurgery* 2010; 67(3), 658-662.

[33] Takagi Y, Kikuta K, Nozaki K, Sawamura K, Hashimoto N. Detection of a residual nidus by surgical microscope-integrated intraoperative near-infrared indocyanine green videoangiography in a child with a cerebral arteriovenous malformation. *J. Neurosurg.* (5 Suppl Pediatrics) 2007; 107, 416-418.

[34] Tanaka T, Kato N, Arai T, Hasegawa Y, Abe T. Surgical Treatment of a Sylvian-Middle Fossa Dural Arteriovenous Fistula Draining into the Basal Vein of Rosenthal with Frontotemporal Craniotomy. *J. Stroke Cerebrovasc. Dis.* 2012; 21(4), 333-337.

[35] Thompson BG, Doppman JL, Oldfield EH. Treatment of cranial dural arteriovenous fistulae by interruption of leptomeningeal venous drainage. *J. Neurosurg.* 1994; 80, 617-623.

[36] Tsutsumi S, Yasumoto Y, Ito M, Oishi H, Arai H, Yoritaka A. Atypical Dural Arteriovenous Fistula Associated with Meningitis. *Neurol. Med. Chir.* (Tokyo) 2008; 48, 68-71.

[37] van Dijk JMC, terBrugge KG, Willinsky RA, Wallace MC. Clinical Course of Cranial Dural Arteriovenous Fistulas With Long-Term Persistent Cortical Venous Reflux. *Stroke.* 2002; 35(5), 1233-1236.

[38] Weil AG, McLaughlin N, Denis D, Bojanowski MW. Tentorial branch of the superior cerebellar artery. *Surg. Neurol. Int.* 2011;2:71.

[39] Woitzik J, Horn P, Vajkoczy P, Schmidek P. Intraoperative control of extracranial-intracranial bypass patency by near-infraredindocyanine green videoangiography. *J. Neurosurg*. 2005; 102, 692-698.

[40] Woitzik J, Peña-Tapia PG, Shneider UC, Vajkoczy P, Thomé C. Cortical perfusion measurement by indocyanine-Green videoangiography in patients undergoing hemidraniectomy for malignant stroke. *Stroke*. 2006;37: 1549-1551.

[41] Yamashita K, Ohe N, Yoshimura S, Iwama T. Intracranial Pial Arteriovenous Fistula – Case Report-. *Neurol. Med. Chir.* [Tokyo] 2007; 47:550-554.

In: Fistuals and Fissures
Editors: Dmitri Pavlovich and Sergei Ivanovich
ISBN: 978-1-62618-068-0

Chapter 9

PATHOGENESIS OF PERIANAL FISTULAS IN CROHN'S DISEASE

*A. M. El-Tawil**
Department of surgery, University Hospital
Birmingham, Birmingham, UK

ABSTRACT

Crohn's disease is a chronic inflammatory disorder that can affect any part of the gastrointestinal tract from the mouth to the anus. The disease is characterized by transmural inflammation that can be complicated by the development of fibrotic strictures, perforation, abscess formation, and fistulization. Perianal fistula is a significant clinical sign in cases with Crohn's disease, which may arise from inflamed or infected anal glands (fistula-in-ano) and/or penetration of fissures or ulcers of the rectum or anal canal. Transmural extension and gut flora play crucial role in the progress and development of Crohn's anal fistulas. The retrieved Escherichia Coli strains from Crohn's disease patients are able to adhere to and to invade intestinal epithelium. They are then capable to survive digestion by the submucosal neutrophils and macrophages.

Persistent infection in Crohn's anal fistulas is mainly due to overproduction of IL-1, IL-6 and TNFα, which are produced by activated macrophages, to poor response to IL-4 and to lack of production of IL-10. This overproduction is further enhanced by the availability of free zinc and the then overproduction of interferon gamma. This likely explains the failure of the concomitant antibiotics Ciprofloxacin for 12 weeks in 24 patients to improve the response to infliximab.

Cyclosporine, Tacrolimus, Azathioprine and 6- Mercaptopurine were all used in treating Crohn's anal fistulas but the outcome was not so successful as it was with infliximab. This is likely because that these thiopurines are mainly acting against activated T Lymphocytes and its productions which play less important role than those produced by activated macrophages.

Although IL-10 is zinc-dependent the provision of zinc would add no benefit. Recombinant IL-10 may offer better chances for better rates of success.

---

* A. M. El-Tawil: Department of surgery, University Hospital Birmingham, 7th Floor, Area 3, Mindelsohn Way, Birmingham. B15 2WB. United Kingdom, E-mail: atawil20052003@yahoo.co.uk.

Keywords: Anal Fistula, Crohn's disease, Infliximab, Thiopurines, Macrophages, Escherichia. Coli, TNF, IL-1, IL-4, IL-6, IL-10, and Interferon gamma

INTRODUCTION

Fistulas occur in 14-26% of patients with Crohn's disease [1-5]. Perianal fistulas comprise half of all cases [3 and 6], whereas enteroenteric comprise 25%, recto/anovaginal comprise 10% and other fistulas (enterocutaneous and enterovesical) account for 10-15% of fistulas in these patients [3 and 6]. Two-thirds of patients experience just one fistula episode, while the remainder have two or more fistula episodes over 20 years of follow-up [3]. In approximately 10% of patients, perianal fistulization is the initial manifestation of Crohn's disease [4] And the formation of perianal fistulas may precede the onset of Crohn's disease by several years [4] Patients with colonic Crohn's disease, particularly those with rectal involvement, have a significantly higher incidence of perianal fistulas than patients without colonic involvement. Perianal fistulas can be further classified as low (located below the dentate line), high (located above the dentate line), simple (low and painless, with a single external opening and no evidence of rectovaginal involvement or anorectal stricture), [7] or complex (located high, can be associated with pain, can potentially involve multiple external openings, a rectovaginal fistula, an anorectal stricture, or active inflammatory rectal disease, as assessed by endoscopy) [8] The presence of a fistula usually indicates a more aggressive course of Crohn's disease, which may include a need for more frequent hospitalizations, surgery, and steroid treatment [9] Despite of the prevalence of fistulas in patients with Crohn's disease, fistula pathogenesis remains poorly understood. For this reason, we are going to examine the possible predisposing factors and their contribution in the development of this abnormality. During the course of this study, we may be able to answer a question on why infliximab was more successful than thiopurines in treating cases of Crohn's anal fistulae and higher significant rates of complete healing of anal fistulae were achieved with the first than with the second regimen.

1. INFECTING AGENTS AND FISTULAE DEVELOPMENT

The first step in the formation of a fistula is generally assumed to be tissue destruction. The transmural inflammation that characterizes Crohn's disease predisposes these patients to fistula formation. Luminal bacteria may also have a role in the development and maintenance of fistulas. Evidence exists to support that the most prevalent bacteria in patients with Inflammatory Bowel Disease are Enterobacteriaceae, especially Escherichia coli [10-12].

The conducted prospective study by Eykyn and Grace in 1986 [13] evidently provides the most informative data on the causative agents in cases with perianal fistulae. The participant patients had an initial examination under anesthesia and a further examination, one week later, by an experienced surgeon to inspect the presence of a fistula. This clinical assessment was harmonized by an enormously inclusive microbiological survey. The significant microbiological findings are summarized in Table 1. Table 1 provides an objective evidence to support the idea that gram negative bacteria are mainly responsible for the development of fistulae in those with anal abscess.

The occurrence of pathogenic Escherichia coli in the large bowel of subjects with Crohn's disease and ulcerative colitis in comparison with control subjects was further examined in a prospective study [14] The findings were then linked to clinical and laboratory measures for finding a correlation. E. coli gene fimA encoding the surface properties was found to be the most frequent gene that occurred in all the investigated groups, including the control subjects. All subjects with the E. coli gene fimA were found to have increased serum IL-6 levels (p=0.05) All subjects carrying the E. coli gene fimA were found to have significant high values of TNF-α (p<0.01) Patients with CD were found to have significantly higher serum level of IL-6 than those with UC (p<0.01) TNF-α was the highest in the UC group (p<0.01). High levels of TNF-α levels were also found in CD but the figures were less than those in UC and mildly higher than those in the control group [14].

The recovered Escherichia Coli strains from patients with Crohn's disease were able to adhere and to invade intestinal epithelial cells. [15-22] When the behaviour within macrophages of adherent invasive *E. coli* (AIEC) strains isolated from patients with CD was analysed all the 15 tested AIEC strains were able to replicate extensively within J774-A1 cells (the numbers of intracellular bacteria increased 2.2- to 74.2-fold at 48 h over that at 1 hour Post-infection. [15] By use of murine peritoneal macrophages and human monocyte-derived-macrophages, the reference AIEC strain LF82 was confirmed to be able to survive intracellularly No lactate dehydrogenase (LDH) release, no sign of DNA fragmentation or degradation, and no binding to fluorescein isothlocyanate-labeled annexin V were observed with LF82-infected J774-A1 cells after 24 h post-infection [15] LF82-infected J774-A1 cells secreted 2.7-fold more tumour necrosis factor alpha (TNF-a) than cells stimulated with 1 mg of lipopolysaccharide (LPS)/ml. No release of interleukin-1b was observed with LPS-pre-stimulated J774-A1 cells infected with AIEC LF82 [15].

Table 1. Type of organisms isolated from anorectal abscesses with and without fistulae

Type of organism	fistula present (n=53)	No fistula (n=27)	
Number of abscesses yielding anaerobes	49 (92.5%)	8 (29.6%)	P<0.0001
Escherichia coli	45 (84.9%)	5 (18.5%)	P<0.0001
Staph. aureus	† 1 (1.9%)	8 (29.6%)	P=0.0012
Anaerobes 'Gut-specific Bacteroids	47 (88.7%)	5 (18.5%)	P<0.0001
Anaerobes not 'gut-specific' (only)	2 (3.8%)	17 (63%)	P<0.0001
Gut aerobes+ 'gut-specific anaerobes'	45 (85%)	4 (14.8%)	P<0.0001

Includes E. coli, Klebsiella spp, Proteus spp, Citrobacter spp, Salmonella sp, Str. faecalis. † Only 2 colonies isolated. (Eykyn, S. J., Grace, R. H. Ann. R Coll Surg. Engl. 1986 Sep;68(5):237-9).

2. Cytokines in Inflammatory Bowel Disease

Cytokines are small peptide molecules of between 5 and 50 k Da, which can be expressed by a number of different cell lineages, but which are most commonly associated with cells of the immune system The majority of these molecules are released as inactive precursors containing a signal peptide, which is then cleaved to give the mature protein.

Certain molecules, such as IL-1, IL-6, TNFα and the chemokines, are predominantly synthesized and released by activated macrophages. IL-1 and IL-6 have the capacity to stimulate both arms of the immune response by activating T cells to produce IL-2 and express the IL-2 receptor, and also by inducing B-cell proliferation, maturation and increased immunoglobulin synthesis.

TNFα similarly has an important role in the inflammatory response and in host resistance, with its ability to induce or suppress expression of a number of genes. These include genes for growth factors and cytokines, transcription factors, receptors, inflammatory mediators and acute phase proteins.

The other major cytokines, which include IL-2, IL-4, IL-5, IL_10, IL-13 and γ interferon are predominantly synthesized and released by activated T lymphocytes. This group of cytokines is further divided into two subgroups because of their different actions and effects on the immune response: (1) The Th1 group, which includes: IL-2 and γ interferon and (2) the Th2, which includes: IL-4, IL-5, IL-10 and IL-13. The Th1 subgroup directs a cell-mediated immune response, whereas the Th2 cytokines generate a humoral response [23, 24].

IL-1 and IL-6 are minimally expressed in normal tissue but TNF-α may be expressed at a higher level. In view of the large amounts of lipopolysaccharide in the intestinal lumen and bathing the mucosa, the resident immune cells (in particular tissue macrophages) appear to have adapted to the environment and become tolerated to these stimuli. This may explain the founded elevated levels of IL-1B in subjects with active Crohn's disease and active ulcerative colitis due to the attribution of mucosal macrophages [25] The concentrations of IL-6 are similarly elevated in active disease, but some studies have shown more significant increase, in patients with Crohn's disease compared with those with ulcerative colitis [26].

A recent report gives in –vitro evidence to suggest that there is an impaired response to IL-4 by activated mononuclear phagocytes in Inflammatory Bowel Diseases [27].

These experiments revealed that both peripheral blood and intestinal phagocytes from patients with Inflammatory Bowel Disease showed a diminished response to the down regulatory effects of IL-4, such as inhibition of IL-1 and TNF production, superoxide anion generation and elevation of IL- 1RA/IL-1 ratio. The study included both normal controls and cases with diverticulitis. [27].

In another study, it was found that the collected lamina proprial Lymphocytes from subjects with active Crohn's disease spontaneously produce IL-2 but no IL-10, whereas cells from patients with ulcerative colitis and controls produced only IL-10 [It is worth to note that both IL-4 and IL-10 could inhibit IL-2-induced synthesis of IFN-gamma and tumour necrosis factor (TNF)-alpha by human peripheral blood mononuclear cells [28 and 29]].

These results may be due to genetic abnormalities. Evidence exists from genetically engineered "knock out" animal models in which a cytokine gene has been deleted. The IL-2 Knock out develops an ulcerative colitis-type disease with inflammation limited to the colon, [30] whereas a IL-10 knock out develops a more widespread enterocolitis [31].

3. Zinc Deficiency and Steroid Sex Hormones and Pro-Inflammatory Cytokines

Reduced plasma zinc concentration is common in Inflammatory Bowel Diseases [32- 48], which may indicate reduced zinc absorption [41, and 49] or increased zinc losses [50 and 51] Zinc urinary output increased significantly after exercise in Crohn's disease patients and remained unchanged in control subjects [51].

Om and Chung (1996) [52] investigated the effects of zinc deficiency on hepatic androgen metabolism and aromatisation, androgen and oestrogen receptor binding, and circulating levels of reproductive hormones in freely fed, pair-fed and zinc-deficient rats. Hepatic conversion of testosterone to dihydrotestosterone was significantly less, but formation of oestradiol from testosterone was considerably higher in rats fed with zinc deficient diet compared with freely fed and pair-fed control rats. There were noticeably lower serum concentrations of lutenising hormone, oestradiol and testosterone in rats fed with zinc deficient diet. Scatchard analyses of the receptor binding data showed a significantly higher level of oestrogen receptors in zinc deficient rats. It is worthy to note that unbound receptors are sensitive to inactivation by dephosphorylation, whereas the oestrogen-bound receptors are unaffected. Phosphorylation- dephosphorylation mechanism is dependent on the existence of zinc [53].

It has been estimated that Lipopolysaccharide could activate pro-inflammatory cytokines by activating plasma membrane proteins (e.g. the toll like receptor 4 [TLR4] and CD14 that leads to the production of TNF and other pro-inflammatory cytokines). In monocytes stimulated with heat-killed *Escherichia coli*, progesterone increased the secretion of IL-1B and the neutrophil chemotactant IL-8 but depressed TNF secretion. [54] Progesterone, estradiol and testosterone, individually reduced the secretion of IL-6 from LPS-activated cells [55] but estradiol and progesterone, together reduced monocyte secretion of IL-1α and IL-1β [56].

4. Zinc, Zinc Finger Proteins, and Cytokines

IL-10 is a potent anti-inflammatory and immunosuppressive cytokine that inhibits a broad spectrum of dendritic cell and macrophage functions, thus effectively limiting the ability of APCs to activate T cells. IL-10 induces down-regulation of MHC class II and the co-stimulatory molecules CD80 and CD86 on APCs [57], in addition to repressing production of the pro-inflammatory cytokines IL-1, IL-6, IL-12, and TNF-α in these cells [57]. In vivo studies have shown $CD4^+$ T cell-derived IL-10 to be critical for restraint of the adaptive immune response and also as an essential mediator of intestinal homeostasis [58]. Although IL-10-deficient mice have enhanced resistance to pathogens compared with wild-type mice, infections can result in the development of host tissue injury, severe immune-mediated disease, and the overproduction of pro-inflammatory cytokines due to uncontrolled effector responses [59-62].

For many of the genes encoding proteins involved in the transport, storage, and function of the trace elements, expression is regulated by the availability of the elements concerned.

This control is exercised through a variety of mechanisms, including metal-activated transcription factors, modified usage of stop codons, and use of secondary structure within mRNA to regulate its translation and stability. Two widely represented groups of transcription factors, often classed as zinc-finger proteins, depend on constituent zinc ions for their activity [63].

Ikaros is a zinc finger DNA-binding protein. It plays an important role in the regulation of *IL-10* in murine $CD4^+$ T cells. Ikaros plays a critical role in activation of *IL-10* expression in $CD4^+$ T cells. Ikaros null T cells are unable to express IL-10 either in a naive state or under Th2 conditions [64].

Yet, it was reported that zinc and micronutrients treatment increased the lymphocyte ratios of CD4 to CD8 and of CD4 CD45RA toCD4 CD45RO, increased the ex vivo generation of interleukin-2 (IL-2) and interferon (IFN), decreased the generation of interleukin-10 (IL-10), and increased plasma interleukin-1 receptor antagonist (sIL-1ra) and soluble tumour necrosis factor receptor 1 (sTNF-R1) in children with zinc deficiency. [65] But micronutrients alone increased the ratio of CD4 to CD8 but not of CD4 CD45RA to CD4CD45RO, increased IFN but had no effect on IL-2 or IL-10, and increased sIL-1ra but not sTNF-R1 [65].

The reported increased production of interferon gamma (IFN) is likely to be due to the availability of free zinc [66] and the resultant overproduction of IFN affected the liberation of IL-10 [67] The effects of IFN-gamma on IL-10 expression in LPS-stimulated monocytes, and the relationship between IL-10 and TNF-alpha production in these cells were examined in an experimental study [67]. The investigators reported that LPS stimulation induced rapid, ordered expression of multiple cytokines. Steady-state mRNA levels for TNF-alpha increased rapidly, reached maximal levels by 2 to 3 h post-stimulation, and then declined sharply. IL-1 beta and IL-6 mRNA levels also increased markedly following stimulation with LPS, but decreased more slowly than did TNF-alpha. Down-regulation of mRNA for TNF-alpha, IL-1 beta, and IL-6 coincided with a delayed and more gradual increase in IL-10 mRNA levels. Furthermore, neutralization of IL-10 with anti-IL-10 Abs prolonged TNF-alpha mRNA expression, and significantly increased net TNF-alpha production. IFN-gamma suppressed expression of IL-10 mRNA and protein in a dose-dependent manner. Moreover, inhibition of IL-10 production correlated with a marked increase in both the magnitude and duration of TNF-alpha expression. This means that potentiating TNF-alpha production by IFN-gamma in monocytes is coupled to inhibition of endogenous IL-10 expression.

Discussion

Fistulizing perianal Crohn's disease is often refractory. It is thus requiring a combination of medical and surgical therapy. Antibiotics [68-72], azathioprine [72, 73], 6-mercaptopurine [74, 75], cyclosprorine [78, 79], and tarcolimus [79] have all demonstrated limited efficacy in published reports. But in 1999, a randomized controlled trial found that infliximab was significantly better than placebo in healing fistulae in Crohn's disease [80] Recent published reports examining infliximab in treating fistulising Crohn's disease have shown complete healing rates of 24 -55 % [81-84] Complete healing rates for perianal fistulae range from 47-56% [84, 85].

Infliximab is a murine chimeric monoclonal antibody against TNF α. Yet, the reason for the persistence of infection in fistulising Crohn's disease is due to the overproduction of IL-1, IL-6, and TNF α by the activated macrophages, poor response to IL-4 and the lack of production of IL-10. This explains the high rates of complete healing with the use of infliximab in this group of patients than with the use of immunosuppressive drugs (Thiopurines are mainly acting against activated T lymphocytes. But as we explained above, IL-2 and interferon gamma in fistulising Crohn's disease play supportive role to the other cytokines but not the main role in fistulising Crohn's disease. This also explains why concomitant antibiotics Ciprofloxacin 500 mg twice per day for 12 weeks in 24 patients did not improve the response to infliximab [86].

REFERENCES

[1] Schwartz, D. A., Loftus, E. V., Jr., Tremaine, W. J., et al. The natural history of fistulizing Crohn's disease in Olmsted County, Minnesota. *Gastroenterology* 2002; 122:875-880.

[2] Lapidus, A. Crohn's disease in Stockholm County during 1990- 2001: an epidemiological update. *World J. Gastroenterol*. 2006; 12:75-81.

[3] Tang, L. Y., Rawsthorne, P., Bernstein, C. N. Are perineal andluminal fistulas associated in Crohn's disease? A population based study. *Clin. Gastroenterol. Hepatol.* 2006; 4:1130-1134.

[4] Hellers, G., Bergstrand, O., Ewerth, S., Holmstrom, B. Occurrence and outcome after primary treatment of anal fistulae in Crohn's disease. *Gut*; 1980; 21:525–527.

[5] Farmer, R. G., Hawk, W. A., Turnbull, R. B., Jr Clinical patterns in Crohn's disease: a statistical study of 615 cases. *Gastroenterology*. 1975;68(4 Pt 1):627–635.

[6] Ingle, S. B., Loftus, E. V., Jr. The natural history of perianal Crohn's disease. *Dig. Liver Dis*. 2007; 39:963-969.

[7] Sandborn, W. J., Present, D. H., Isaacs, K. L., Wolf, D. C., Greenberg, E., Hanauer, S. B., Feagan, B. G., Mayer, L., Johnson, T., Galanko, J., Martin, C., Sandler, R. S. (2003) Tacrolimus for the treatment of fistulas in patients with Crohn's disease: a randomized, placebo-controlled trial. *Gastroenterology* 125: 380–388

[8] American Gastroenterological Association Clinical Practice Committee (2003) American Gastroenterological Association medical position statement: perianal Crohn's disease. *Gastroenterology* 125: 1503–1507

[9] Nielsen, O. H., Rogler, G., Hahnloser, D., et al. Diagnosis and management of fistulizing Crohn's disease. *Nat. Clin. Pract. Gastroenterol. Hepatol.* 2009;6:92-106.

[10] Guarner, F., Malagelada, J. R. Role of bacteria in experimental colitis. *Best Pract. Res. Clin. Gastroenter*ol. 2003 Oct.;17(5):793-804.

[11] El-Tawil, A. M._High incidence of Crohn's disease in pre-menopausal women: Escherichia coli may be contributing. *Int. J. Colorectal. Dis*. 2004 Sep.; 19(5):498.

[12] Rolhion, N. and Darfeuille-Michaud, A. Adherent-Invasive Escherichia coli in Inflammatory Bowel Disease. *Inflamm. Bowel Dis*. 2007;13:1277–12783)

[13] Eykyn, S. J., Grace, R. H. The relevance of microbiology in the management of anorectal sepsis. *Ann. R Coll Surg. Engl.* 1986 Sep.; 68(5):237-9.

[14] Gombošová, L., Lazúrová, I., Zakuciová, M., Čurová, K., Kmeťová, M., Petrášová, D., and Siegfried, L. Genes of intestinal Escherichia coli and their relation to the inflammatory activity in patients with ulcerative colitis and Crohn's disease. *Folia Microbiol.* (2011) 56:367–372

[15] Glasser, A. L., Boudeau, J., Barnich, N., Perruchot, M. H., Colombel, J. F., Darfeuille-Michaud, A. Adherent invasive Escherichia coli strains from patients with Crohn's disease survive and replicate within macrophages without inducing host cell death. *Infect. Immun.* 2001 Sep.; 69(9):5529-37

[16] Darfeuille-Michaud, A., Neut, C., Barnich, N., Lederman, E., Di Martino, P., Desreumaux, P., Gambiez, L., Joly, B., Cortot, A., Colombel, J. F. Presence of adherent Escherichia coli strains in ileal mucosa of patients with Crohn's disease. *Gastroenterology*. 1998 Dec.; 115(6):1405-13

[17] Chassaing, B., Rolhion, N., de Vallée, A., Salim, S. Y., Prorok-Hamon, M., Neut, C., Campbell, B. J., Söderholm, J. D., Hugot, J. P., Colombel, J. F., Darfeuille-Michaud, A. Crohn disease--associated adherent-invasive E. coli bacteria target mouse and human Peyer's patches via long polar fimbriae. *J. Clin. Invest.* 2011 Mar.; 121(3):966-75.

[18] Barnich, N., Carvalho, F. A., Glasser, A. L., Darcha, C., Jantscheff, P., Allez, M., Peeters, H., Bommelaer, G., Desreumaux, P., Colombel, J. F., Darfeuille-Michaud, A. CEACAM6 acts as a receptor for adherent-invasive E. coli, supporting ileal mucosa colonization in Crohn disease. *J. Clin. Invest.* 2007 Jun.;117(6):1566-74

[19] Rolhion, N., Darfeuille-Michaud, A. Adherent-invasive Escherichia coli in inflammatory bowel disease. *Inflamm. Bowel Dis.* 2007 Oct.; 13(10):1277-83.

[20] Bringer, M. A., Rolhion, N., Glasser, A. L., Darfeuille-Michaud, A. The oxidoreductase DsbA plays a key role in the ability of the Crohn's disease-associated adherent invasive Escherichia coli strain LF82 to resist macrophage killing. *J. Bacteriol.* 2007 Jul.; 189(13):4860-71.

[21] Barnich, N., Bringer, M. A., Claret, L., Darfeuille-Michaud, A. Involvement of lipoprotein NlpI in the virulence of adherent invasive Escherichia coli strain LF82 isolated from a patient with Crohn's disease. *Infect. Immun.* 2004 May;72(5):2484-93.

[22] Boudeau, J., Glasser, A. L., Masseret, E., Joly, B., Darfeuille-Michaud, A. Invasive ability of an Escherichia coli strain isolated from the ileal mucosa of a patient with Crohn's disease. *Infect. Immun.* 1999 Sep.; 67(9):4499-509.

[23] Mosmann, T. R., Coffman, R. L. TH1 and TH2 cells: different patterns of lymphokine secretion lead to different functional properties. *Annu. Rev. Immunol.* 1989;7:145-73.

[24] Maggi, E., Parronchi, P., Manetti, R., Simonelli, C., Piccinni, M. P., Rugiu, F. S., De Carli, M., Ricci, M., Romagnani, S._Reciprocal regulatory effects of IFN-gamma and IL-4 on the in vitro development of human Th1 and Th2 clones *J. Immunol.* 1992 Apr. 1;148(7):2142-7

[25] Mahida, Y. R., Ceska, M., Effenberger, F., Kurlak, L., Lindley, I., Hawkey, C. J. Enhanced synthesis of neutrophil-activating peptide-1/interleukin-8 in active ulcerative colitis. *Clin. Sci.* (Lond.) 1992 Mar.; 82(3):273-5.

[26] Mitsuyama, K., Sata, M., Tanikawa, K._Significance of interleukin-6 in patients with inflammatory bowel disease *Gastroenterol. Jpn.* 1991 Feb.; 26(1):20-8.

[27] Schreiber, S., Heinig, T., Panzer, U., Reinking, R., Bouchard, A., Stahl, P. D., Raedler, A. Impaired response of activated mononuclear phagocytes to interleukin 4 in inflammatory bowel disease *Gastroenterology*. 1995 Jan.; 108(1):21-33

[28] Hsu, D. H., Moore, K. W., Spits, H. Differential effects of IL-4 and IL-10 on IL-2-induced IFN-gamma synthesis and lymphokine-activated killer activity. *Int. Immunol.* 1992 May;4(5):563-9

[29] Schreiber, S., Heinig, T., Thiele, H. G., Raedler, A. Immunoregulatory role of interleukin 10 in patients with inflammatory bowel disease *Gastroenterology.* 1995 May;108(5):1434-44

[30] Sadlack, B., Merz, H., Schorle, H., Schimpl, A., Feller, A. C., Horak, I. Ulcerative colitis-like disease in mice with a disrupted interleukin-2 gene. *Cell.* 1993 Oct. 22;75(2):253-61

[31] Kühn, R., Löhler, J., Rennick, D., Rajewsky, K., Müller, W. Interleukin-10-deficient mice develop chronic enterocolitis. *Cell.* 1993 Oct. 22;75(2):263-74.

[32] Solomons, N. W., Rosenberg, I. H., Sandstead, H. H., Vo-Khactu, K. P. Zinc deficiency in Crohn's disease. *Digestion* 1977; 16:87–95.

[33] Tasman-Jones, C. Zinc deficiency states. *Adv. Intern. Med.* 1980; 26:97–114.

[34] Fleming, C. R., Huizenga, K. A., McCall, J. T., Gildea, J., Dennis, R. Zinc nutrition in Crohn's disease. *Dig. Dis. Sci.* 1981; 26:865–870.

[35] Sandstead, H. H., Howard, L., Zinc deficiency in Crohn's disease. *Nutr. Rev.* 1982; 40:109–112.

[36] Fagerlund, T. H., Dahl, D. G. Zinc deficiency as a complication of Crohn disease. *Tidsskr. Nor. Laegeforen* 1983; 103:999–1000.

[37] Penny, W. J., Mayberry, J. F., Aggett, P. J., Gilbert, J. O., Newcombe, R. G., Rhodes, J Relationship between trace elements, sugar consumption, and taste in Crohn's disease. *Gut* 24 1983;288–292.

[38] Deflandre, J., Weber, G., Delbrouck, J. M., Roelandts, I., Robaye, G., Brassinne, A. Assay of trace elements in the serum by the PIXE method in patients with Crohn's disease. *Gastroenterol. Clin. Biol.* 1985; 9:719–725.

[39] McClain, C. J. Zinc metabolism in malabsorption syndromes. *J. Am. Coll. Nutr.* 1985; 4:49–64.

[40] Steinberg, S. E. Zinc deficiency in Crohn's disease. *Compr. Ther.* 1985; 11:34–38.

[41] Valberg, L. S., Flanagan, P. R., Kertesz, A., Bondy, D. C. Zinc absorption in inflammatory bowel disease. *Dig. Dis. Sci.* 1986; 31:724–731.

[42] Hendricks, K. M., Walker, W. A. Zinc deficiency in inflammatory bowel disease. *Nutr. Rev.* 1988; 46:401–408.

[43] Sjo¨gren, A., Flore´n, C. H., Nilsson, A. Evaluation of zinc status in subjects with Crohn's disease. *J. Am. Coll. Nutr.* 1988; 7:57–60.

[44] Geerling, B. J., Badart-Smook, A., Stockbru¨gger, R. W., Brummer, R. J. Comprehensive nutritional status in patients with long-standing Crohn disease currently in remission. *Am. J. Clin. Nutr.* 1998; 67:919–926.

[45] Matsui, T. Zinc deficiency in Crohn's disease. *J. Gastroenterol.* 1998; 33:924–925.

[46] Naber, T. H., van den Hamer, C. J., Baadenhuysen, H., Jansen, J. B. The value of methods to determine zinc deficiency in patients with Crohn's disease. *Scand. J. Gastroenterol.* 1998;33:514– 523.

[47] Ojuawo, A., Keith, L. The serum concentrations of zinc, copper and selenium in children with inflammatory bowel disease. *Cent. Afr. J. Med.* 2002;48:116–119.

[48] Schu¨tz, T., Drude, C., Paulisch, E., Lange, K. P., Lochs, H. Sugar intake, taste changes and dental health in Crohn's disease. *Dig. Dis.* 2003; 21:252–257.

[49] Griffin, I. J., Kim, S. C., Hicks, P. D., Liang, L. K., Abrams, S. A. Zinc metabolism in adolescents with Crohn's disease. *Pediatr. Res.* 2004; 56:235–239.

[50] Stoll, R., Schmidt, H., Stern, H., Ruppin, H., Domschke, W. Functional defect of zinc transport in patients with Crohn's disease. *Hepatogastroenterology* 1987; 34:178–181.

[51] D'Inca,` R., Varnier, M., Mestriner, C., Martines, D., D'Odorico, A., Sturniolo, G. C. Effect of moderate exercise on Crohn's disease patients in remission. *Ital. J. Gastroenterol. Hepatol.* 1999; 31:205–210

[52] Om, A. S., Chung, K. W. (1996) Dietary zinc deficiency alters 5 alpha-reduction and aromatization of testosterone and androgen and estrogen receptors in rat liver. *J. Nutr.* 126:842–848.

[53] Nielsen, C. J., Sando, J. J., Pratt, W. B. (1977) Evidence that dephosphorylation inactivates glucocorticoid receptors. *Proc. Natl. Acad. Sci. US* 74:1398–1402.

[54] Peltier, M. R., Tee, S. C., Smulian, J. C._Effect of progesterone on proinflammatory cytokine production by monocytes stimulated with pathogens associated with preterm birth. *Am. J. Reprod. Immunol.* 2008 Oct.;60(4):346-53.

[55] Jain, S. K., Kannan, K., Prouty, L., Jain, S. K._Progesterone, but not 17beta-estradiol, increases TNF-alpha secretion in U937 monocytes. *Cytokine.* 2004 May 7;26(3):102-5.

[56] Morishita, M., Miyagi, M., Iwamoto, Y._Effects of sex hormones on production of interleukin-1 by human peripheral monocytes. *J. Periodontol.* 1999 Jul.; 70(7):757-60.

[57] Wun, K. S., Cameron, G., Patel, O., Pang, S. S., Pellicci, D. G., Sullivan, L. C., Keshipeddy, S., Young, M. H., Uldrich, A. P., Thakur, M. S., et al. A molecular basis for the exquisite CD1d-restricted antigen specificity and functional responses of natural killer T cells. *Immunity.* 2011;34:327–339

[58] Jayawardena-Wolf, J., Benlagha, K., Chiu, Y. H., Mehr, R., Bendelac, A. CD1d endosomal trafficking is independently regulated by an intrinsic CD1d-encoded tyrosine motif and by the invariant chain. *Immunity.* 2001;15:897–908.

[59] Bezbradica, J. S., Stanic, A. K., Matsuki, N., Bour-Jordan, H., Bluestone, J. A., Thomas, J. W., Unutmaz, D., Van Kaer, L., Joyce, S. Distinct roles of dendritic cells and B cells in Va14Ja18 natural T cell activation in vivo. *J. Immunol.* 2005;174:4696–4705.

[60] Griewank, K., Borowski, C., Rietdijk, S., Wang, N., Julien, A., Wei, D. G., Mamchak, A. A., Terhorst, C., Bendelac, A. Homotypic interactions mediated by Slamf1 and Slamf6 receptors control NKT cell lineage development. *Immunity.* 2007;27:751–762.

[61] Park, S-H., Roark, J. H., Bendelac, A. Tissue specific recognition of mouse CD1 molecules. *J. Immunol.* 1998;160:3128–3134.

[62] Liu, Y., Goff, R. D., Zhou, D., Mattner, J., Sullivan, B. A., Khurana, A., Cantu, C., 3rd, Ravkov, E. V., Ibegbu, C. C., Altman, J. D., et al. A modified alpha-galactosyl ceramide for staining and stimulating natural killer T cells. *J. Immunol. Methods.* 2006;312:34–39.

[63] Chesters, J. K. Trace element-gene interactions. *Nutr. Rev.* 1992 Aug.; 50(8):217-23.

[64] Umetsu, S. E. and Winandy, S. Ikaros Is a Regulator of *Il10* Expression in $CD4^+$ T Cells. *J. Immunol.* 2009 November 1; 183(9): 5518-5525.

[65] Sandstead, H. H., Prasad, A. S., Penland, J. G., Beck, F. W., Kaplan, J., Egger, N. G., Alcock, N. W., Carroll, R. M., Ramanujam, V. M., Dayal, H. H., Rocco, C. D., Plotkin, R. A., Zavaleta, A. N._Zinc deficiency in Mexican American children: influence of zinc and other micronutrients on T cells, cytokines, and antiinflammatory plasma proteins. *Am. J. Clin. Nutr.* 2008 Oct.;88(4):1067-73.

[66] Bao, B., Prasad, A. S., Beck, F. W., Bao, G. W., Singh, T., Ali, S., Sarkar, F. H. Intracellular free zinc up-regulates IFN-γ and T-bet essential for Th1 differentiation in Con-A stimulated HUT-78 cells. *Biochem. Biophys. Res. Commun.* 2011 Apr. 22;407(4):703-7

[67] Donnelly, R. P., Freeman, S. L., Hayes, M. P._Inhibition of IL-10 expression by IFN-gamma up-regulates transcription of TNF-alpha in human monocytes. *J. Immunol.* 1995 Aug. 1;155(3):1420-7.

[68] Ursing, B., Kamme, C. Metronidazole for Crohn's disease. *Lancet.* 1975 Apr. 5;1(7910):775-7.

[69] Bernstein, L. H., Frank, M. S., Brandt, L. J., Boley, S. J. Healing of perineal Crohn's disease with metronidazole. *Gastroenterology*. 1980 Sep.; 79(3):599.

[70] Brandt, L. J., Bernstein, L. H., Boley, S. J., Frank, M. S. Metronidazole therapy for perineal Crohn's disease: a follow-up study. *Gastroenterology*. 1982 Aug.; 83(2):383-7.

[71] Jakobovits, J., Schuster, M. M. Metronidazole therapy for Crohn's disease and associated fistulae. *Am. J. Gastroenterol.* 1984 Jul.; 79(7):533-40.

[72] Dejaco, C., Harrer, M., Waldhoer, T., Miehsler, W., Vogelsang, H., Reinisch, W. Antibiotics and azathioprine for the treatment of perianal fistulas in Crohn's disease. *Aliment Pharmacol. Ther.* 2003 Dec.; 18(11-12):1113-20.

[73] Rhodes, J., Bainton, D., Beck, P., Campbell, H. Controlled trial of azathioprine in Crohn's disease. *Lancet.* 1971 Dec. 11;2(7737):1273-6.

[74] Korelitz, B. I., Present, D. H. Favorable effect of 6-mercaptopurine on fistulae of Crohn's disease. *Dig. Dis. Sci.* 1985 Jan.; 30(1):58-64.

[75] Markowitz, J., Rosa, J., Grancher, K., Aiges, H., Daum, F. Long-term 6-mercaptopurine treatment in adolescents with Crohn's disease. *Gastroenterology.* 1990 Nov.; 99(5):1347-51.

[76] Mahadevan, U., Marion, J. F., Present, D. H. Fistula response to methotrexate in Crohn's disease: a case series. *Aliment Pharmacol. Ther.* 2003 Nov. 15;18(10):1003-8.

[77] Present, D. H., Korelitz, B. I., Wisch, N., Glass, J. L., Sachar, D. B., Pasternack, B. S. *N Engl. J. Med.* 1980 May 1;302(18):981-7.

[78] Hanauer, S. B., Smith, M. B. Rapid closure of Crohn's disease fistulas with continuous intravenous cyclosporin A. *Am. J. Gastroenterol.* 1993 May; 88(5):646-9.

[79] Lowry, P. W., Weaver, A. L., Tremaine, W. J., Sandborn, W. J. Combination therapy with oral tacrolimus (FK506) and azathioprine or 6-mercaptopurine for treatment-refractory Crohn's disease perianal fistulae. *Inflamm. Bowel Dis.* 1999 Nov.; 5(4):239-45.

[80] Present, D. H., Rutgeerts, P., Targan, S., Hanauer, S. B., Mayer, L., van Hogezand, R. A., Podolsky, D. K., Sands, B. E., Braakman, T., DeWoody, K. L., Schaible, T. F., van Deventer, S. J. Infliximab for the treatment of fistulas in patients with Crohn's disease. *N Engl. J. Med.* 1999 May 6;340(18):1398-405.

[81] Cohen, R. D., Tsang, J. F., Hanauer, S. B. Infliximab in Crohn's disease: first anniversary clinical experience. *Am. J. Gastroenterol.* 2000 Dec.; 95(12):3469-77.

[82] Sample, C., Bailey, R. J., Todoruk, D., Sadowski, D., Gramlich, L., Milan, M., Cherry, R., Ma, M., Lalor, E., McKaigney, J., Sherbaniuk, R., Matic, K., Switzer, C., Fedorak, R. N. Clinical experience with infliximab for Crohn's disease: the first 100 patients in Edmonton, Alberta. *Can. J. Gastroenterol.* 2002 Mar.; 16(3):165-70.

[83] Arnott, I. D., McDonald, D., Williams, A., Ghosh, S. Clinical use of Infliximab in Crohn's disease: the Edinburgh experience. *Aliment Pharmacol. Ther.* 2001 Oct.; 15(10):1639-46.

[84] Ricart, E., Panaccione, R., Loftus, E. V., Tremaine, W. J., Sandborn, W. J. Infliximab for Crohn's disease in clinical practice at the Mayo Clinic: the first 100 patients. *Am. J. Gastroenterol.* 2001 Mar.; 96(3):722-9.

[85] Farrell, R. J., Shah, S. A., Lodhavia, P. J., Alsahli, M., Falchuk, K. R., Michetti, P., Peppercorn, M. A. Clinical experience with infliximab therapy in 100 patients with Crohn's disease. *Am. J. Gastroenterol.* 2000 Dec.; 95(12):3490-7.

[86] West, R. L., van der Woude, C. J., Hansen, B. E., Felt-Bersma, R. J., van Tilburg, A. J., Drapers, J. A., Kuipers, E. J. Clinical and endosonographic effect of ciprofloxacin on the treatment of perianal fistulae in Crohn's disease with infliximab: a double-blind placebo-controlled study. *Aliment Pharmacol. Ther.* 2004 Dec.; 20(11-12):1329-36.

In: Fistuals and Fissures
Editors: Dmitri Pavlovich and Sergei Ivanovich
ISBN: 978-1-62618-068-0

Chapter 10

SETONS IN TREATMENT OF ANAL FISTULA

Gokulakkrishna Subhas*
Providence Hospital and Medical Centers, Southfield, MI, US

ABSTRACT

High trans-sphincteric fistulas, involving the upper two-thirds of the external sphincter, remain a surgical challenge because incontinence may result from the division of muscle involving more than one-third of the sphincter. The principles of anal fistula surgery are to eliminate the fistula, prevent recurrence and preserve sphincter function.

In contrast with fistulotomy for low anal fistulas, a well-accepted, simple, safe, and efficient method is still lacking for high anal fistulas. Seton techniques still occupy an important position in the treatment of high anal fistulas. The seton works by several mechanisms: (1) it helps in draining pus and controlling sepsis prior to definitive treatment; (2) it stimulates fibrosis and acts as a marker of the fistula tract for sphincter sparing procedures such as fistula plug, fibrin glue and ligation of intersphincteric fistula tract (LIFT); and (3) the tight (cutting) seton promotes slow transection of the external sphincter muscle as a result of pressure necrosis with minimal separation of the cut ends.

Long-term seton drainage is a simple and efficient procedure in treating high anal fistulas in Crohn's disease. This article describes the current options available for management of anal fistula with setons. When a patient presents with anal fistula, it is important to determine the level of fistula, involvement of sphincters (high vs low transphincteric), abscess or local sepsis and the etiology. For low fistula involving less than a third of the sphincters, primary fistulotomy can be performed. For high transphincteric fistula with abscess and local sepsis, a loose seton to act as drainage seton or a drainage tube seton should be placed. Once the abscess has resolved than for a crypt glandular fistula the treatment decision involves the use of sphincter sparing vs sphincter cutting options. Setons for such treatment can be considered either as a cutting or loose seton after discussing the individual merits with the patients. Cutting seton can be used as a single stage or multi-stage procedure. Currently cutting setons are not in much use in the developed countries because of the pain associated with treatment, uncontrolled cutting of sphincter muscles and a higher rate of incontinence. If the patient is willing to try for a prolonged treatment option then he can be offered the long term loose seton. For

* E-mail: drsgokul@yahoo.com.

patients who want to opt for sphincter saving surgery the loose setons are generally left in the fistula tract for 4-6 weeks. Also patient who had started on long term loose seton, but did not want to continue with loose seton, can be considered for one of the sphincter sparing surgery.

Patients with Crohn's disease have a higher risk of recurrence. Once the perianal sepsis is controlled with loose drainage setons/ drainage tubes, consideration should be given for treatment with biological agents such as infliximab. After the disease and sepsis is under control these patient can choose between long term loose seton or sphincter sparing surgeries.

Introduction

Anal fistula is believed to originate from an infection of the anal glands. Fistula-in-ano is a common complex disease process. The majority of perianal fistulae are low fistulae which include the submucous, intersphincteric, and most of the transsphincteric types of anal fistula. [1] The object of surgical treatment of an anal fistula is to eradicate it without disturbing anal continence. These goals can be achieved by laying open (fistulotomy) or excising the fistulous tract (fistulectomy) in an intersphincteric or low transsphincteric fistula.

However, laying open a high transsphincteric, suprasphincteric or extrasphincteric fistula involves division of most, or all, of the sphincter muscle, which would compromise continence. [2] Setons play an important role in the treatment of high anal fistulas. Seton division is an old surgical process which is still widely applied for the management of complex fistula problems. It is a relatively simple technique with a universally accepted good cure rate. [3]

The word seton is derived from the Latin word 'Seta' meaning bristle and it refers to any foreign material inserted through the fistulous tract. [4] The Indian surgeon Sushruta is first credited with describing the use of a chemical seton in the treatise Sushruta Samhita (600 BC). Hippocrates (460-377 BC) advocated a cutting seton method consisting of 'horsehair wrapped about a lint thread' which was advanced through the fistula with a tin guide; the ends of this seton were then tied around the enclosed sphincter tissue and tightened at periodic intervals 'until the flesh was eaten through'. Albucasis in the 11th century described a two stage seton technique wherein he inserted a seton following fistulotomy. A modification of this technique was described by John of Arderne in his Treatise on the cure of fistula in 1376. Dittel in Vienna reported the use of India rubber ligature in the treatment of fistula. William Allingham of St Mark's Hospital, London published his experience of 60 cases of anal fistula with elastic seton in 1875. [4] Different materials and techniques have since been used for treating anal fistula. [5] Setons have been described for the treatment of fistula-in-ano in infants with favorable results. [6]

Fistula Types

There have been different classification systems for anal fistula. The classification system described by Parks is the most commonly used classification system. When it comes to treatment decision making, the most important factor is the amount sphincter muscles below the fistula tract. Some authors have described high fistula is one in which a limb or track of the fistula passes above the highest muscle of continence (the anorectal ring or puborectalis muscle). [7]

Mechanism of Action of Seton

The seton works by several mechanisms: (1) It assists in identifying and marking the fistula tract during excision of a trans-sphincteric fistula; (2) it helps in draining pus and controlling sepsis prior to definitive treatment; (3) it stimulates fibrosis to prevent retraction of the cut ends of the external sphincter, following delayed division for completion of fistulotomy; (4) the tight (cutting) seton promotes slow transaction of the external sphincter muscle; (5) the long term loose seton used specially in patients with Crohn's disease helps in controlling perineal sepsis. [8]

Other simpler way to look at the principle of a seton conceptually, is that it can be used as a marker or a divider. [9] When a seton is used as a marker, the entire fistulous tract may be encircled without dividing any portion of the sphincter muscle. Seton are used as a marker in staged fistulotomy in which the cephalad half of the sphincter mechanism is divided in a controlled fashion and a seton is left to mark the site of the remaining fistulous tract, thus converting a high fistula into a low fistula.

Setons are used a marker in the sphincter sparing fistula repair wherein the presence of fistula will promote fibrosis around the tract and make identification and handling of fistula tract easier during the surgery. Seton acts as a divider of the sphincter muscles in tight cutting setons and also in some of the long term loose setons. [10]

Figure 1. helps in decision making with regards to setons choice for the treatment of fistula.

Cutting Setons

One of the traditional managements of high trans-sphincteric fistula-in-ano, where the fistula tract passes through more than half of the external and internal anal sphincter musculature, has been the use of the cutting seton. The advantages of such a technique include its ability to drain the region with the prevention of recurrent abscesses, the promotion of fibrosis around the seton (which in theory will prevent retraction of the continence musculature behind its advancement) and the capacity to serve as a landmark for the fistula during delayed fistulotomy or fistulectomy. [11]

In the cutting seton technique, the seton is used to strangulate the intervening tissues so that the sphincters are slowly transected. Initially a tight seton is placed in the fistulous track around the anal sphincter and tied with tension. The seton is then tightened at different intervals of time as required until the sphincter mechanism was transected. [12] A cutting seton works by slowly transecting the enclosed sphincter muscle as a result of pressure necrosis with minimal separation of the cut ends.

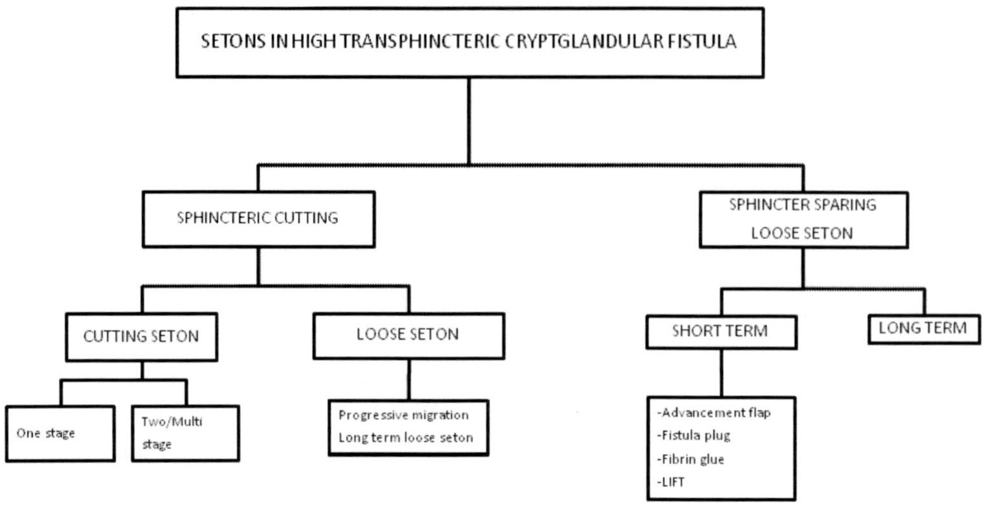

Figure 1. Setons in high transphincteric fistula.

Classically, a silk suture or other foreign material is inserted through the complex fistulous tract and intermittently tightened. [13] Seton's application in the management of high anal fistula is based on the assumption that a chronic inflammatory reaction is caused thereby stimulating fibrosis. This fixes and prevents retraction and separation of sphincter muscle when it is divided in order to protect the sphincter continuity during the procedure. This process may be considered similar to that of a wire cutting a block of ice slowly, where the ice is still adherent after the division. [3]

Appropriate static tension of the seton pulled around the external sphincter assures the success of treatment. The use of too much tension may result in discomfort for patients, whereas it is impossible to cut the sphincter if the seton is tied too loosely. The maintenance and regulation of static tension is often a great problem. [14]

Staged Fistulotomy

Two-stage seton fistulotomy is a widely practiced method which utilizes the seton to mark the tract and stimulate fibrosis, followed by delayed incision of the sphincters as a second procedure. This method is, by definition, a staged procedure, and it is not free from significant disturbances in anal continence. [13] Seton is used as part of a staged fistulotomy in which the cephalad half of the sphincter mechanism is divided in a controlled fashion and a seton is left to mark the site of the remaining fistulous tract, thus converting a high fistula into a low fistula. After the cephalad portion of the sphincter has healed, so that the anorectal ring has reformed, the remaining low fistulous tract can be divided safely. Some authors believe that the staged fistulotomy using a seton as a guide is preferable to the progressive tightening of a seton to slice through the sphincter muscle. As the latter procedure may inflict unnecessary pain on the patient because it pinches and abrades the edematous anoderm. Also, this uncontrolled method of dividing the sphincter may be unsuccessful if the muscle is too thick or may lead to pressure necrosis of the full thickness of the sphincter muscle, resulting in sepsis, fecal incontinence, or both. This "piecemeal" fistulotomy is usually performed in two stages, but, if an extraordinarily large amount of the sphincter mechanism is involved in a high fistula, the surgeon should not hesitate to perform the procedure in three or more stages. The second-stage fistulotomy should be carried out six to eight weeks after the first to allow for adequate healing of the cephalad portion of the sphincter and to re-establish continuity of the anorectal ring, In most instances, second- stage fistulotomy with removal of the intact seton can be handled in an outpatient setting using local anesthesia. [9]

Cutting seton versus two-stage seton fistulotomy in the surgical. Both techniques are equally effective in eradicating the fistula, and both are associated with a similar rate of incontinence. [15]

NEWER FISTULA TREATMENTS

The approach by the coloproctologist towards complex recurrent high fistula-in-ano should be individually based on his or her experience and judgement. It is probably unwise to use cutting setons in patients who already have impaired continence before surgery, or in multiparous women with high anterior trans-sphincteric fistulas. [11] Anal fistula treatment has evolved to include a variety of noncutting techniques in addition to traditional fistulotomy. With the advent of more sphincter-sparing techniques, the number of patients undergoing fistulotomy should continue to decrease over time. The fibrin sealant technique involves the closure of fistula tract using fibrin glues which are a combination of thrombin and fibrinogen. An anal fistula plug is an acellular porcine submucosal collagen designed to allow growth of fibroblasts into its scaffolding. This plug when placed in the fistula tract helps in closure of fistulas. An endorectal advancement flap is a flap of rectal wall including mucosa, submucosal, and superficial smooth muscle which is raised cephalad. The primary opening of the fistula is closed and the flap is brought down and sutured to the anoderm. Ligation of the intersphincteric fistula tract (LIFT) is performed by an incision which is made parallel to the anal verge and deepened, separating the internal and external sphincters until the fistula tract is encountered. An indwelling probe facilitates identification of the tract. The tract is then encircled, ligated at both the proximal and distal ends with absorbable sutures, and the fistula tract is divided with or without excision of a segment of the tract. Surgeons should become familiar with various surgical techniques so the treatment can be tailored to the patient. [16]

For all these newer techniques, the initial treatment involves placement of a loose seton for a period of about four to six weeks. This loose seton helps in drainage and sepsis control, promotes fibrosis around the tract and acts as a marker of the tract during definitive surgery.

VARIATIONS IN MATERIALS, TECHNIQUES

There are many seton techniques in use in current surgical practice, including chemical setons, drainage setons, cutting setons, and two-stage seton fistulotomy. However, the pros and cons of different seton techniques have not been clearly established. [3, 5] A variety of materials have been used: suture, stainless steel wire, depezzar catheters, medicated ksharsootra, self-locking cable, silicone, thread, and rubber bands. Hollow 3-mm diameter silastic tube seton allowing the clear visualization of drained fistula tracks with MRI have been described as well. [17] After intraoperative rectal evaluation and placement of the seton, several methods have been used to progressively tighten the seton. Patients are sometimes asked to re-tie it tighter. The seton can be removed in the office and another placed more snugly. Ligiclips can be placed progressively proximally. A rubber band ligator can be used in a similar fashion. Descriptions have been made using the hangman's tie and self-locking cable tie. While being effective, these methods can be technically unrewarding as the area is unclean, not easily accessible, and local excoriation is frequently encountered. There has to be a good balance between maintaining the appropriate tension while preventing perianal pressure necrosis The mean cut-out time varies between days and 6 months and is related to the tension on the seton, fistula complexity, and associated underlying pathology. [18]

Techniques have been described with marsupialization after fistulotomy. Marsupialization after anal fistula surgery is postulated to leave less raw unepithelialized tissue in the fistulotomy (or fistulectomy) wound thereby resulting in less postoperative blood loss and faster wound healing. [19] Postoperatively, warm sitz baths after each bowel movement were advised. The patients were informed in detail about the presence of the setons, and they were warned about the possible serous discharge that would continue until the seton dropped. [13]

Long-term seton drainage will not result in fistula healing, but drainage of sepsis prevented further abscesses. [20] The long term suture ensures a continuous drainage of the fistula, and daily bowel movements also cause a moderate pull on the suture, resulting in the fistula gradually but continually becoming shorter. The procedure is visible through the increase in length of the suture. The suture either "cuts through" the anal and perianal skin on its own after a suitable period, i.e., the fistula recedes fully, or the remaining fistula is lanced in an operation. This method, whereby the suture is tied loosely and remains in place for a long period of time, is essentially different from other setons in which one or more sutures are tied under tension. [21]

The 'permanent loose seton' technique may be considered the treatment of choice in the majority of Crohn's disease patients, as it is effective in preventing local sepsis in many patients over time and is associated with a low complication rate. [22] The loose seton approach is efficacious as a definitive long-term treatment for primary high trans-sphincteric anal fistula in cases of persistence or recurrence even non-Crohn's etiology. [8] In case of high transphincteric fistula, loose seton are used with the aim of external anal sphincter preservation, allowing drainage of sepsis and maturation of tracts. Such drainage of sepsis allowed clearer delineation of the fistula tract and safer definitive surgery. [23]

CROHNS DISEASE

Asymptomatic fistulas in patients with Crohn's disease need not be treated. Symptomatic fistulas and abscesses require therapy. Fistulotomy has been associated with poor wound healing, recurrent sepsis, incontinence, and proctectomy. The technique of long-term, indwelling setons functioning as drains was developed in an effort to prevent or delay proctectomy. The technique is not difficult and requires only the ability to accurately identify the primary opening. [24]

Perianal fistulas occur in up to 30 percent of patients with Crohn's disease. They often are recurrent, complex, and associated with ongoing perianal sepsis. The literature presents opposing views on the role of surgery in the treatment of this difficult condition. Fistulotomy is argued to be safe in superficial fistulas; however, incontinence rates of up to 50 percent are reported. There also has been concern expressed that fistulotomy may aggravate anal lesions, which in up to 40 percent of patients, fail to heal. Moreover many perianal Crohn's fistulas are high, complex fistulas. An alternative method of symptom control is long-term indwelling seton drainage. [25] Long-term seton drainage is a simple and efficient procedure in treating high anal fistulas in Crohn's disease. Once inserted, seton allows primary eradication of sepsis in about 70 percent of cases, and incontinence caused by the technique itself rarely occurs[26]

Setons are reported to prevent recurrent suppuration. However, the recurrence of perianal sepsis with the seton in situ is still reported to be between 23 and 44 percent. Long-term indwelling seton is an effective management modality for complex perianal Crohn's fistulas and seems to decrease the need for temporary or permanent stomas. [25]

Recurrence and Incontinence

The guiding principle of the surgical elimination of perianal fistulae is complete removal of the fistular passage on the one hand, and the sparing of the sphincteric musculature of the anus (avoidance of incontinence). Furthermore, that operation technique should be applied that helps avoid recurrences. [27] Interestingly, a great variability of continence impairment after seton placement has been published, ranging from 0% to 70%. [12] The recurrence rate following treatment with cutting setons is reported to be 2%–8% in the literature. The reported rate of total continence disorders is about 60%; flatus incontinence, 36.2%; liquid stool incontinence, 8.5%; and solid stool incontinence, 2.3%. [28]

Although complete division and healing of the sphincter mechanism using a seton seldom result in total incontinence, minor control problems occur in many patients. The degree of incontinence is probably related to the patient's preoperative state of anal control as well as how precisely the anal wound heals. If the edges of the fistulotomy wound do not approximate precisely, or if an inordinate amount of scar tissue develops, small gaps may persist or the anus may not be able to close properly, which would lead to intermittent leakage of gas or liquid stool. Special consideration should be given to elderly patients or those individuals who have undergone prior anorectal fistulotomy or lateral internal sphincterotomies since these factors may compromise the integrity of the sphincter mechanism. Further division of the external sphincter muscle in these patients should be carried out with caution or after careful manometric examination. [9]

Conclusion

An anal fistula is an affliction that tests the patience of the surgeon and the patient alike. Setons play an important role in the treatment of high anal fistula. Approaching the fistulas with the intent to cure, the surgeon must always keep in mind the fine balance between an aggressive approach resulting in cure and incontinence and a conservative approach, preserving continence and resulting in recurrence or persistence and the need for additional operative procedures. In case of patients with Crohn's disease and chronic perianal sepsis, drainage setons should be considered during active abscess and sepsis which should be followed by loose setons. After the disease and sepsis is under control and the patient does not want to continue with loose seton, then consideration can be given for the sphincter sparing surgery. Surgeons should be aware of the newer sphincter sparing surgeries and these options should be discussed with the patients.

REFERENCES

[1] Theerapol, A., B.Y. So, and S.S. Ngoi, Routine use of setons for the treatment of anal fistulae. *Singapore medical journal*, 2002. 43(6): p. 305-7.

[2] Williams, J.G., et al., Seton treatment of high anal fistulae. *The British journal of surgery*, 1991. 78(10): p. 1159-61.

[3] Chuang-Wei, C., et al., Cutting seton for complex anal fistulas. *The surgeon: journal of the Royal Colleges of Surgeons of Edinburgh and Ireland*, 2008. 6(3): p. 185-8.

[4] McCourtney, J.S. and I.G. Finlay, Setons in the surgical management of fistula in ano. *The British journal of surgery*, 1995. 82(4): p. 448-52.

[5] Subhas, G., et al., Setons in the Treatment of Anal Fistula: Review of Variations in Materials and Techniques. *Digestive surgery*, 2012. 29(4): p. 292-300.

[6] Ikeda, T., et al., Treatment of fistula-in-ano in infants with a seton. *Journal of pediatric surgery*, 2007. 42(6): p. 1095-7.

[7] Parks, A.G. and R.W. Stitz, The treatment of high fistula-in-ano. *Diseases of the colon and rectum*, 1976. 19(6): p. 487-99.

[8] Eitan, A., M. Koliada, and A. Bickel, The use of the loose seton technique as a definitive treatment for recurrent and persistent high trans-sphincteric anal fistulas: a long-term outcome. *Journal of gastrointestinal surgery: official journal of the Society for Surgery of the Alimentary Tract*, 2009. 13(6): p. 1116-9.

[9] Pearl, R.K., et al., Role of the seton in the management of anorectal fistulas. *Diseases of the colon and rectum*, 1993. 36(6): p. 573-7; discussion 577-9.

[10] Subhas, G., et al., Non-cutting setons for progressive migration of complex fistula tracts: a new spin on an old technique. *International journal of colorectal disease*, 2011. 26(6): p. 793-8.

[11] Zbar, A.P., et al., Conventional cutting vs. internal anal sphincter-preserving seton for high trans-sphincteric fistula: a prospective randomized manometric and clinical trial. *Techniques in coloproctology*, 2003. 7(2): p. 89-94.

[12] Vial, M., et al., Faecal incontinence after seton treatment for anal fistulae with and without surgical division of internal anal sphincter: a systematic review. *Colorectal disease: the official journal of the Association of Coloproctology of Great Britain and Ireland*, 2010. 12(3): p. 172-8.

[13] Mentes, B.B., et al., Elastic one-stage cutting seton for the treatment of high anal fistulas: preliminary results. *Techniques in coloproctology*, 2004. 8(3): p. 159-62.

[14] Dziki, A. and M. Bartos, Seton treatment of anal fistula: experience with a new modification. *The European journal of surgery = Acta chirurgica,* 1998. 164(7): p. 543-8.

[15] Garcia-Aguilar, J., et al., Cutting seton versus two-stage seton fistulotomy in the surgical management of high anal fistula. *The British journal of surgery*, 1998. 85(2): p. 243-5.

[16] Blumetti, J., et al., Evolution of treatment of fistula in ano. *World journal of surgery*, 2012. 36(5): p. 1162-7.

[17] Armstrong, T., et al., Hollow seton for magnetic resonance imaging fistula visualization. *Colorectal disease: the official journal of the Association of Coloproctology of Great Britain and Ireland*, 2006. 8(7): p. 615.

[18] Awad, M.L., H.W. Sell, and K.R. Stahlfeld, Split-shot sinker facilitates seton treatment of anal fistulae. *Colorectal disease: the official journal of the Association of Coloproctology of Great Britain and Ireland*, 2009. 11(5): p. 524-6.

[19] Malik, A.I. and R.L. Nelson, Surgical management of anal fistulae: a systematic review. *Colorectal disease: the official journal of the Association of Coloproctology of Great Britain and Ireland*, 2008. 10(5): p. 420-30.

[20] Joy, H.A. and J.G. Williams, The outcome of surgery for complex anal fistula. *Colorectal disease: the official journal of the Association of Coloproctology of Great Britain and Ireland*, 2002. 4(4): p. 254-261.

[21] Lentner, A. and V. Wienert, Long-term, indwelling setons for low transsphincteric and intersphincteric anal fistulas. Experience with 108 cases. *Diseases of the colon and rectum*, 1996. 39(10): p. 1097-101.

[22] Galis-Rozen, E., et al., Long-term outcome of loose seton for complex anal fistula: a two-centre study of patients with and without Crohn's disease. *Colorectal disease: the official journal of the Association of Coloproctology of Great Britain and Ireland*, 2010. 12(4): p. 358-62.

[23] Davies, M., et al., The surgical management of fistula-in-ano in a specialist colorectal unit. *International journal of colorectal disease*, 2008. 23(9): p. 833-8.

[24] White, R.A., et al., Seton management of complex anorectal fistulas in patients with Crohn's disease. *Diseases of the colon and rectum*, 1990. 33(7): p. 587-9.

[25] Thornton, M. and M.J. Solomon, Long-term indwelling seton for complex anal fistulas in Crohn's disease. *Diseases of the colon and rectum*, 2005. 48(3): p. 459-63.

[26] Faucheron, J.L., et al., Long-term seton drainage for high anal fistulas in Crohn's disease--a sphincter-saving operation? *Diseases of the colon and rectum*, 1996. 39(2): p. 208-11.

[27] Balogh, G., Tube loop (seton) drainage treatment of recurrent extrasphincteric perianal fistulae. *American journal of surgery*, 1999. 177(2): p. 147-9.

[28] Vatansev, C., et al., A new seton type for the treatment of anal fistula. *Digestive diseases and sciences*, 2007. 52(8): p. 1920-3.

In: Fistuals and Fissures
Editors: Dmitri Pavlovich and Sergei Ivanovich

ISBN: 978-1-62618-068-0

Chapter 11

BILIARY FISTULAS

Elham Dadzan, Chirag S. Desai and Raffaele Girlanda
Georgetown University Hospital, Department of Surgery,
Washington DC, US

ABSTRACT

Biliary fistulas are uncommon but important causes of significant morbidity and mortality, especially in the elderly patient. The classification of biliary fistulas and the clinical scenarios presented by patients with biliary fistulas have changed over the last two decades following the widespread application of operations on the biliary tract, from laparoscopic cholecystectomy to advanced hepato-biliary surgery to liver transplantation. In addition, there has been a dramatic expansion of non-surgical treatment modalities for biliary disease from both the endoscopic and interventional radiology approach. As a result, these new treatment modalities have not only remarkably improved the treatment of biliary disease, but also introduced new complications, including biliary fistulas, which have been recently described. Early recognition and prompt management of biliary fistulas are essential steps for an effective treatment and to reduce mortality. In addition, the treatment of chronic underlying infection and the maintenance of an adequate nutritional support are critical steps in the management of these often debilitated patients. In this review we present an updated classification of biliary fistulas based on current pathophysiology and describe the different clinical scenarios presented by patients with biliary fistulas. We also emphasize key aspects in the multidisciplinary approach to these patients and highlight current diagnostic and treatment strategies.

INTRODUCTION

A fistula is defined as an abnormal communication between a hollow viscus and the skin (external fistula) or another internal organ (internal fistula). Biliary fistulas include all pathological tracts communicating between the biliary tree and the skin or other organs.

Although an uncommon entity, biliary fistulas are a cause of significant morbidity and mortality (Dadzan 2012).

Elderly patients are especially at high risk of complications and mortality from biliary fistulas, given the higher incidence of complicated biliary tract disease in advanced age including gallstone disorders. In addition to old age, other risk factors for complicated biliary disease and biliary fistulas are obesity and diabetes. Recently, the dramatic increase in operative instrumentation on the biliary tract following the introduction of laparoscopic cholecystectomy as the standard treatment for gallstone disease and the continuous expansion of the surgical indications for the treatment of advanced cancer of the biliary tract have resulted in increased risk of post-operative biliary fistula. Furthermore, recent progress in the non-surgical approach to biliary tract disease in high risk patients, including endoscopic and percutaneous interventional radiologic techniques, have opened new clinical scenarios that were largely unknown a couple of decades ago in terms of treatment options and the associated treatment-related complications. As a result of recent advances in the management of biliary tract disease, the number, types and presentations of biliary fistulas have dramatically changed compared to a couple of decades ago. In this chapter we present an updated classification of biliary fistulas along with their pathophysiology and principles of current management.

Definition

A biliary fistula is an abnormal communication between the biliary tract (gallbladder, bile duct, or the liver) and the surface of the body (*external* biliary fistula) or an internal organ (*internal* biliary fistula, see below).

Epidemiology

Fistulas as a complication of gallstones disease used to be more common in the past; nowadays biliary fistulas have become less common following the widespread treatment of gallstones. Indeed, laparoscopic cholecystectomy for the treatment of gallstones has now become one of the most commonly performed abdominal operations. As a result, clinicians have now become less familiar with the presentation and management of biliary fistulas as complications of gallstone disease. However, since many more operations and instrumentations of the biliary tract are now being performed compared to a couple of decades ago, the associated risk of complications has also increased, giving origin to a potentially increasing incidence of "iatrogenic" biliary fistulas (see below).

Classification

Biliary fistulas are classified in a) *external* if they communicate the biliary tract with the external surface of the body or b) *internal* when they involve the abdominal or thoracic cavity and/or an internal organ. They are further characterized by the anatomic denomination of the structure involved. All structures and organs adjacent to the liver and the biliary tract are potentially involved by a biliary fistula (see figure 1).

A) External Biliary Fistula

External biliary fistulas are more common than internal fistulas and usually result as complications of biliary surgery, liver surgery including liver resections or instrumentation of the biliary tract ("iatrogenic") or following abdominal trauma. They are classified in controlled when the bile is drained outside the abdominal cavity or uncontrolled when bile collects in the abdominal cavity and contaminates the peritoneal surfaces resulting in localized or diffuse biliary peritonitis.

Laparoscopic cholecystectomy is currently one of the most commonly performed abdominal operations. Although it has become now a very safe treatment of gallstones, complications include biliary fistulas, biliary strictures and biliary obstructions. The incidence of biliary fistula after laparoscopic cholecystectomy has been extimated around 1% (de Palma 2002). In the majority of cases the bile leak originates from the stump of the cystic duct. Less frequently the leak is from ducts of Lutscka or from the common hepatic duct. A risk factor for bile leak after cholecystectomy is the presence of retained common bile duct stone or papillary stenosis, resulting in increased pressure in the biliary tree. The treatment of choice is usually endoscopic sphincterotomy with or without positioning of naso-biliary drainage or biliary stent in order to decompress internally the biliary tract. A percutaneous drainage of intra-abdominal bile collections is indicated in presence of large leaks. The endoscopic and percutaneous treatment is effective in virtually all cases without need for re-operation (Singh 2010).

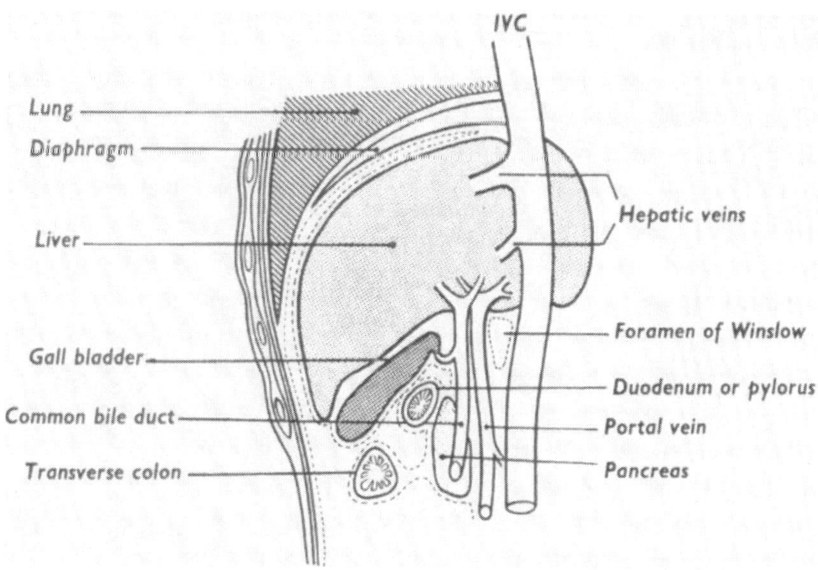

Reproduced from: Spontaneous internal biliary fistulae, Dowse JL, Gut 1964;5: 429-36 with permission from BMJ Publishing Group Ltd.

Figure 1. Diagram showing the close proximity of the extrahepatic biliary tree to adjacent organs target of biliary fistula.

Biliary fistula is also a complication of partial hepatectomy with an incidence reported between 3 and 23% in differect clinical series (Hoekstra 2012, Li 2009). Risk factors include major liver resections, repeat liver resection, prolonged operative time and relaparotomy. The presence of a variant biliary anatomy has also been recognized as a risk factor for unrecognized biliary injury and subsequent bile leak after liver resection and segmental liver transplantation (Jassem 2008). The treatment is usually conservative with percutaneous aspiration of bile collections and endoscopic sphincterotomy with insertion of biliary stent, which leads to resolution of the bile leak in more than 90% of cases (Battacharya 2003, Coelho-Prabhu 2012). In patients who underwent biliary reconstruction with Roux-en-Y hepatico-jejunostomy the percutaneous trans-hepatic biliary drainage is the approach of choice to decompress the biliary tract and to allow the bile leak to seal in the majority of cases.

Less commonly biliary fistula are secondary to abdominal trauma involving the liver, especially in patients with high grade traumatic liver injury (Bala 2012).

Rarely, a spontaneous external biliary fistula has been reported as a complication of chronic calcolous cholecystitis (Ijaz 2008). This fistula, presenting with a right upper quadrant abscess, is now exceptionally unusual given the common institution of antibiotic therapy and early surgery for gallstones disorders. Other unusual cases of external biliary fistula have been reported including cholecysto-cutaneous fistula involving the right breast (Andersen 2012) or the gluteal region (Nicholson 1999).

B) Internal Biliary Fistula

Internal biliary fistulas are less common than external biliary fistulas but they have been known to complicate chronic gallstones disease since the 1950s (review in Dowse 1964). The incidence of internal biliary fistula is difficult to estimate from the many small series reported in the literature. Duzgun *et al* report an incidence of 0.3% of internal biliary fistulas found during cholecystectomy (Duzgun 2007). In other studies the reported incidence of bilio-enteric fistula diagnosed at the time of cholecystectomy is 1-1.2 %% (Dorrance 1999, Leung 2010). Most internal biliary fistulas are diagnosed intraoperatively during cholecystectomy and often require conversion from laparoscopic to open approach.

Unlike external biliary fistulas that are usually iatrogenic or traumatic, internal biliary fistulas are more frequently spontaneous and often diagnosed incidentally during investigations or operations for unrelated conditions.

Internal fistulas involve the duodenum, colon, stomach and common bile duct, in decreasing order of frequency (see Figure 1). The most common cause of internal biliary fistula is gallstones (90%); uncommon causes include peptic ulcer disease, gallbladder cancer, abdominal trauma to the right upper quadrant, hepatobiliary infections and congenital anomalies of the biliary tract. In patients with gallstones, the formation of internal biliary fistula is attributed to a mechanism of pressure-necrosis and erosion of the biliary tract by a solitary impacted stone against adjacent structures, often following bouts of inflammation, infection or obstruction.

Patients with biliary enteric fistula may have symptoms similar to those with chronic cholecystitis and cholelithiasis or other non-specific symptoms related to the upper gastro-intestinal tract. The diagnosis is often made during cholecystectomy. The diagnosis should also be considered whenever air is demonstrated within the biliary system on roentgenographic examination (pneumobilia). However, the presence of air in the biliary tree is nonspecific. A previous bilio-enteric anastomosis, infection, gas-containing gallstones, neoplasia, trauma, an incompetent sphincter of Oddi and congenital anomalies have been implicated as factors in the production of pneumobilia. An additional test to confirm the presence of an internal biliary fistula is a barium study, which outlines the stomach, duodenum and small intestine and demonstrates the passage of barium into the gallbladder or the ductal system through a fistula. A failure to demonstrate a fistula by this procedure could be an indication for a barium enema. Alternatively, endoscopy may also reveal a fistula. The most common internal biliary fistulas are cholecysto-duodenal and cholecysto-colic. Here we describe the following internal biliary fistulas: cholecysto-duodenal fistula including Bouveret syndrome, cholecysto-colonic fistula, cholecysto-choledocal fistula including Mirizzi syndrome, gallstones ileus and the rare internal biliary fistula involving the pleural cavity or the bronchial tree.

Cholecysto-duodenal and Bouveret Syndrome

This is the commonest type of bilio-enteric fistula (70%). A fistula between the gallbladder and the duodenum may be diagnosed incidentally during cholecystectomy or present with acute cholecystitis, upper gastro-intestinal bleeding or liver abscess (Stamou 2006). Occasionally, it may be the first presentation of symptoms in the right upper quadrant in patients without known history of gallstones (Chong 2009). Delayed diagnosis, old age, associated comorbidity and sepsis are risk factors for increased mortality.

Bouveret´s syndrome (Bhama 2002) is a rare form of complicated cholecysto-duodenal fistula characterized by duodenal obstruction due to the passage of gallstones from the gallbladder to the duodenum through a cholecysto-duodenal or cholecysto-gastric fistula. Endoscopy is the main diagnostic procedure, allowing visualisation of the stone and often of the fistulous tract. Fragmentation and removal of the stone endoscopically is also a therapeutic option. Other diagnostic studies include plain abdominal film, barium studies, and axial imaging including ultrasound scan and computed tomography. Up to 40% of pts with bilio-enteric fistula have common duct stones, thus requiring endoscopic or surgical duct clearance if symptomatic during or after the treatment for biliary fistula.

Cholecysto-colonic

A fistula between the gallbladder and the colon is the second most common form of bilio-enteric fistula. Like other bilio-enteric fistulas, often it is discovered intra-operatively during procedures for other conditions (review in Costi 2009, Salemis 2009). In symptomatic cases the diagnosis should be suspected in elderly female with chronic diarrhea. Recently it has been reported as a complication of locoregional liver tumor ablation (Pua 2011). The recent increase in percutaneous procedures in the treatment of liver tumours should increase the awareness of the possibility of this complication.

Cholecysto-choledocal and Mirizzi Syndrome

This is the third form of bilio-enteric fistula, often diagnosed during investigations for a biliary cholic (Nguyen 2005). It is also a presentation of a number of abnormalitites and clinical scenarios involving the gallbladder, the cystic duct, the hepatic duct and the duodenum called Mirizzi syndrome (review Beltran 2012).

Mirizzi syndrome includes a number of chronic complications of symptomatic gallstone disease, mainly derived from a pressure ulcer caused by an impacted gallstone at the gallbladder infundibulum. The impacted gallstone causes compression and obstruction of the bile duct, and eventually erodes into the bile duct, resulting in a cholecysto-choledochal or cholecysto-hepatic fistula with different degrees of communication between the gallbladder and bile duct. This complication is currently rare in developed countries with an incidence of less than 1% (Dorrance 2009), but it is more common in developing countries (4-5%). The importance of including Mirizzi syndrome in the differential diagnosis of gallstones-related complications derives by its potential to cause more serious surgical complications including common bile duct injury.

Gallstone Ileus

This is an uncommon complication of gallstones disease characterized by intestinal obstruction caused by a gallstone impacted in the terminal ileum or at the ileocecal valve (review in Ayantunde 2007). The classic triad (Rigler's triad) of pneumobilia, small bowel obstruction and ectopic gallstone on plain abdominal plain film, although present in only a third of cases, should be diagnostic of gallstone ileus. The diagnosis is confirmed by computed tomography in most of the cases. This scenario represents only 1-2% of all causes of small bowel obstruction in patients with gallstones disease, but the incidence is higher in elderly patients. The mechanism of intestinal obstruction is usually due to a single stone that has migrated from the gallbladder to the intestinal lumen via a bilio-enteric fistula. The stone is large enough (2 or 3 cm) to obstruct partially or completely the terminal ileum, usually within the last 50 cm. The typical presentation is unexplained ileus in an elderly patient with known history of gallstones disease. The presence of two of the signs of the triad has been considered pathognomonic and is encountered in 40–50 % of the cases (Clavien 1990). The change of location of a previously observed stone has also been recognized as a diagnostic clue. The management of gallstone ileus, like other obstruction syndromes in the elderly, includes prompt resuscitation and urgent surgical enterolithotomy, because the stone will not pass spontaneously.

Broncho-pleural Biliary Fistula (Review in Liao 2011)

Rarely a biliary fistula develops with either pleural cavity or the bronchial tree. Most of the cases in the developed world are iatrogenic (a complication of percutaneous biliary instrumentation) (Al-Qahtani 2011) or secondary to penetrating trauma (Gandhi 2009). Worldwide, including Mediterranean area, North Africa, Mexico, echinococcal or amebic abscess have been observed to cause bilio-pleuric and bilio-bronchial fistula (Kabiri 2011).

PRINCIPLES OF DIAGNOSIS AND MANAGEMENT

The diagnosis of a biliary fistula is dependent on its mode of presentation. A high index of suspicion should consider the possibility of a biliary fistula in presence of unexplained abdominal pain, fever, cholangitis in an elderly patient with history of gallstones. Other clinical manifestations include right upper quadrant cellulitis or suppuration and right side pleuritic chest pain. Laboratory tests may show leukocytosis and abnormal liver function.

Radiologic imaging plays an important role in the diagnosis and management of biliary fistulas. Plain and contract radiographs may show pneumobilia or reflux of contrast in the biliary tract. Axial imaging (ultrasound, computed tomography, magnetic resonance imaging and cholangiogram) demonstrates the presence, location and extent of a bile leak and delineates the relationship with surrounding organs involved in the fistula. Axial imaging however does not differentiate bile collections from other fluid accumulations, although the usual presentation of a biloma is that of a unilocular, well circumscribed, extraorgan fluid collection. Ultrasound or CT guidance are used for percutaneous drainage of bilomas and in the follow-up to monitor the resolution of the fistula.

Hepatobiliary scintigraphy utilizing hepatoiminodiacetic acid (HIDA) is a sensitive, although nonspecific, test for identifying biliary leaks and fistulas. This imaging modality is currently seldom used due to its limitations of poor resolution compared to modern axial imaging modalities and it cannot always provide precise anatomical localisation of the site of bile leak. It can be helpful in the follow-up of a biloma.

The injection of contrast medium into a fistulous tract or through a surgical drain is able to demonstrate the site of communication with the biliary system, but the presence of debris may limit the delineation of the entire extent of the fistula (Kissin 1987).

The optimal mode of imaging to define the anatomy of a biliary fistula is based on cholangiography, which is able to delineate the location of the fistula and its extent. Cholangiography can be performed endoscopically (endoscopic retrograde cholangiography (ERC), percutaneously (percutaneous transhepatic cholangiogram, PTC) and intra-operatively. The advances in imaging modalities and in minimally invasive interventional techniques over the last two decades have facilitated the non-operative treatment of most cases of biliary fistula.

ERCP usually visualizes the bile leak but may not always fully depict the extent of a biliary fistula especially in presence of a biliary stricture. In addition, ERCP may fail to opacify all of the proximal biliary tree and may not identify anomalous intrahepatic bile ducts. It may also be technically complex, although not impossible, in patients with previous surgery involving the upper gastro-intestinal tract. However, in addition to its diagnostic yeld, the endoscopic approach represents an invaluable treatment modality in the management of iatrogenic bile leaks by insertion of endoscopic stents or nasobiliary tubes, endoprostheses, sphincterotomy, and balloon dilatation of biliary strictures (Ponchon 1989, Hoff 1998).

PTC visualises very well the intra- and extra-hepatic biliary anatomy, although it is often difficult in patients with nondilated bile ducts. Like the endoscopic approach, the transhepatic access has been used not only in the diagnosis but for the treatment of biliary fistulas (Ponchon 1989).

Biliary fistulas may represent complex clinical scenarios that are best managed by a multidisciplinary team of surgeons, interventional radiology and gastroenterology. The overall goal in the management of a patient with biliary fistula is the closure of the fistula and the restoration of normal anatomy. Initially the patient is resuscitated and stabilized with intravenous fluids, antibiotics, correction of electrolytes imbalances and restoration of adequate nutrition. Additional important steps in the initial management of biliary fistula are the drainage of foci of sepsis and the control of fistula drainage and skin care in presence of external fistula. After obtaining appropriate axial imaging and delineation of the anatomy of the biliary fistula, the endoscopic management includes visualization of the location of the fistula and relief of distal biliary obstruction in order to reduce the intraductal biliary pressure. Often, percutaneous drainage of associated subhepatic or subphrenic abscesses is obtained.

The management of patients with external biliary fistula depends on the etiology and on the controlled or uncontrolled nature of the fistula. Usually, post-operative external biliary fistulas are approached endoscopically in the attempt to relief any cause of biliary obstruction. In a patient with uncontrolled fistula percutaneous ultrasound-guided or CT-guided aspiration and drainage is attempted. In case of failed percutaneous control or in unstable patients with diffuce biliary peritonitis, surgical exploration and open drainage is indicated. The goal of surgical exploration and drainage is to establish control of the fistula rather than obtain primary repair of the fistula. Indeed, the majority of fistulas close spontaneously with time provided that there is no obstruction to the bile flow downstream and that bilio-enteric continuity is maintained.

The asymptomatic or mildly symptomatic patient with internal biliary fistula may never require surgical treatment of the fistula. Alternatively, the symptomatic elderly patient may present a too high risk/benefit ratio to consider surgical treatment. Elective surgery in the symptomatic and low risk patient with internal biliary fistula may include pre-operative endoscopic papillotomy with clearance of the common bile duct followed by cholecystectomy and excision of the biliary fistula with exploration of the common bile duct.

The management of gallstones ileus in its classical presentation follows the principles of treatment of intestinal obstruction as a surgical emergency that should only be delayed to allow naso-gastric decompression, fluid resuscitation and stabilization of the patient. The cause of obstruction (impacted stone) is in the terminal ileum in the majority of the cases. The stone is usually mobile in the lumen of the intestine and can be pushed up more proximally to allow an enterotomy and estraction of the stone with primary suture of the intestinal wall.

Conclusion

The presentation of patients with biliary fistula has changed over the last two decades following recent advances in the treatment of multiple benign and malignant conditions involving the biliary tract, from gallstones to cholangiocarcinoma. The morbidity and mortality risk is increased in the elderly patient with associated co-morbidity and in patients with delayed or missed diagnosis. The management of these patients is optimized by a multi-disciplinary approach involving surgeons, gastroenterologists and interventional radiologists.

References

Al-Qahtani H. H. Biliopleural fistula with cholethorax. A rare complication of percutaneous transhepatic biliary drainage. *Saudi Med J.* 2011 Nov; 32 (11):1189-92.

Andersen P., Friis-Andersen H. 2012 Spontaneous cholecystocutaneous fistula presenting in the right breast. *Ugeskr Laeger*. 2012;174:1235-6.

Ayantunde A. A., Agrawal A. Gallstone ileus: diagnosis and management. *World J Surg*. 2007 Jun; 31(6):1292-7.

Bala M., Gazalla S. A., Faroja M., Bloom A. I., Zamir G., Rivkind A. I., Almogy G. Complications of high grade liver injuries: management and outcomewith focus on bile leaks. *Scand J Trauma Resusc Emerg Med.* 2012 Mar 23;20:20.

Beltrán M. A. Mirizzi syndrome: History, current knowledge and proposal of a simplified classification. *World J Gastroenterol* 2012 Sep 14; 18(34): 4639-50.

Bhattacharjya S., Puleston J., Davidson B. R., Dooley J. S. Outcome of early endoscopic biliary drainage in the management of bile leaks after hepatic resection. *Gastrointest Endosc.* 2003 Apr; 57(4):526-30.

Chong V. H., Lim K. S., Mathew V. V. Spontaneous gallbladder perforation, pericholecystic abscess and cholecystoduodenal fistula as the first manifestations of gallstone disease. Hepatobiliary Pancreat Dis Int. 2009 Apr;8(2):212-4.

Coelho-Prabhu N., Nagorney D. M., Baron T. H. ERCP for the treatment of bile leak after partial hepatectomy and fenestration for symptomatic polycystic liver disease. *World J Gastroenterol* 2012;18(28):3705-9.

Costi R., Randone B., Violi V., Scatton O., Sarli L., Soubrane O., Dousset B., Montariol T. Cholecystocolonic fistula: facts and myths. A review of the 231 published cases. *J Hepatobiliary Pancreat Surg.* 2009;16 (1):8-18.

Dadzan E., Akhondi H. Choledochoduodenal fistula presenting with pneumobilia in a patient with gallbladder cancer: a case report. *Journal of Medical Case Reports* 2012 6:61.

de Palma G. D., Galloro G., Iuliano G., Puzziello A., Persico F., Masone S., Persico G. Leaks from laparoscopic cholecystectomy. *Hepatogastroente-rology* 2002 Jul-Aug;49(46): 924-5.

Dorrance H. R., Lingam M. K., Hair A., Oien K., O'Dwyer P. J. Acquired abnormalities of the biliary tract from chronic gallstone disease. *J Am Coll Surg.* 1999 Sep;189 (3):269-73.

Duzgun A. P., Ozmen M. M., Ozer M. V., Coskun F. Internal biliary fistula due to cholelithiasis: a single-centre experience. *World J Gastroenterol.* 2007; 13 (34):4606-9.

Gandhi N., Kent T., Kaban J. M., Stone M., Teperman S., Simon R. Bronchobiliary fistula after penetrating thoracoabdominal trauma: Case report and literature review. *J Trauma.* 2009 Nov;67 (5):E143-5.

Hoekstra L. T., van Gulik T. M., Gouma D. J., Busch OR Posthepatectomy bile leakage: How to manage. *Dig Surg.* 2012;29 (1):48-53.

Hoff W. S., Ginsberg G. G., Grossman M. D., Reilly P. M., Kauder D. R., Schwab C. W. Traumatic choledochogastric fistula: endoscopic evaluation and treatment with a biliary stent. *J Trauma.* 1998 Dec;45 (6):1094-6.

Ijaz S., Lidder S., Mohamid W., Thompson H. H. Cholecystocutaneous fistula secondary to chronic calculous cholecystitis. *Case Rep Gastroenterol.* 2008 Mar 11;2 (1):71-5.

Jassem W., Heaton N. D., Rela M. Reducing bile leak following segmental liver transplantation: understanding biliary anatomy of the caudate lobe. Am J Transplant. 2008 Feb;8 (2):271-4.

Kabiri E. H., Traibi A., Arsalane A. [Bilio-bronchial fistula due to hydatic disease: case report and review of the literature]. *Rev Pneumol Clin.* 2011 Dec;67 (6):380-3.

Kissin C.M., Grundy A. Percutaneous transhepatic cholangiography in the investigation of the persistent postoperative bile leak. *Gastrointest Radiol.* 1987;12 (3):215-8.

Leung E., Kumar P. Bilo-enteric fistula (BEF) at laparoscopic cholecystectomy: review of ten year's experience. *Surgeon* 2010 Apr;8(2):67-70.

Li J., Malagó M., Sotiropoulos G. C., Lang H., Schaffer R., Paul A., Broelsch C. E., Nadalin S. Intraoperative application of "white test" to reduce postoperative bile leak after major liver resection: results of a prospective cohort study in 137 patients. *Langenbecks Arch Surg.* 2009 Nov;394 (6):1019-24.

Liao G. Q., Wang H., Zhu G. Y., Zhu K. B., Lv F. X., Tai S. Management of acquired bronchobiliary fistula: A systematic literature review of 68 cases published in 30 years. *World J Gastroenterol* 2011 Sep 7;17(33):3842-9.

Nguyen D. H., Miller S. D., Robinson E. K., Adler D. G. Cholecystocholedochal fistula. Gastrointest Endosc. 2005 Jun;61 (7):876.

Nicholson T., Born M. W., Garber E. Spontaneous cholecystocutaneous fistula presenting in the gluteal region. *J Clin Gastroenterol* 1999 Apr; 28(3): 276-7.

Ponchon T., Gallez J. F., Valette P. J., Chavaillon A., Bory R. Endoscopic treatment of biliary tract fistulas. *Gastrointest Endosc.* 1989 Nov-Dec;35(6):490-8.

Pua U., Merkle E. M. Case report. Spontaneous cholecystocolic fistula and locoregional liver tumour ablation: a cautionary tale. *Br J Radiol.* 2011 Dec;84 (1008):e243-5.

Schiappa J. M. Iatrogenic lesions of the biliary tract. *Acta Chir Belg.* 2008 Mar-Apr;108 (2):171-85.

Salemis N. S., Georgoulis E., Tsohataridis E. Cholecystocolic fistula: an unusual presentation and review of literature. *Trop Gastroenterol.* 2009 Jul-Sep;30 (3):152-3.

Singh V., Singh G., Verma G. R., Gupta R. Endoscopic management of postcholecystectomy biliary leakage. *Hepatobiliary Pancreat Dis Int.* 2010 Aug;9 (4):409-13.

Stamou K. M., Kekis P. B., Glynatsis M. Gallbladder-duodenal fistula presenting with liver abscess and upper gastrointestinal bleeding. *HPB* (Oxford). 2006;8 (1):69-70.

In: Fistuals and Fissures
Editors: Dmitri Pavlovich and Sergei Ivanovich

ISBN: 978-1-62618-068-0

Chapter 12

ARM FISTULAE AND THEIR CREATION

A. N. Hopper and C. Davies
Morriston Hospital, Wales, UK

ABSTRACT

The autogenous arterio-venous fistula (AVF) is the gold standard in establishing long-term vascular access in end stage renal disease (ESRD) and can be established in the majority of patients as a day case under local anaesthetic. General anaesthesia is typically only required for more complicated, secondary procedures. Pre-operative clinical examination and duplex ultrasonography are essential in planning vascular access procedures and thus maximising the chances of the fistula being useful for long-term dialysis.

It is imperative that "Venous real estate" be utilised in a careful manner. Peripheral veins should be preserved in all patients (especially those at risk of requiring future renal replacement therapy) by avoiding unnecessary venesection or cannulation. Fistulae should be constructed as distally as possible thus maximising the number of sites that can be used. The most distal fistula should be performed preferably in the non-dominant upper limb.

If possible centrally placed double-lumen catheters and prosthetic grafts should be avoided because of their relatively high complication rates. However, both have roles to play in the management of renal failure patients especially in the emergent situation or when autogenous methods are no longer possible.

The snuff-box fistula is an ideal first fistula. It can be constructed in half of all patients and has good patency rates. The construction of this fistula, the brachio-cephalic and transposed brachial vein fistulae are discussed in this chapter.

INTRODUCTION

Chronic access to the vascular system is required for long-term renal replacement therapy (RRT). The ideal properties of this access are listed in Table 1. In the 1960s vascular access was achieved using an extra-corporeal plastic tube tied into a suitable artery and vein (Scribner shunt).

Table 1. Properties of ideal vascular access

Properties
Low infection rate
High primary patency rate
Low failure or revision rate (with high secondary patency rate)
Allow circulation of blood of at least 300ml/minute through a dialysis machine
Sited in non-dominant upper limb (to allow self-needling in home dialysis, or the patient to perform tasks such as reading and writing whilst dialysing)

This was prone to thrombosis and infective complications. The autogenous arterio-venous fistula (AVF) was introduced in the late 1960s by Cimino and Brescia and remains the gold standard in establishing long-term vascular access in end stage renal disease (ESRD) to this day. The shunt allows a high flow of blood with relatively low thrombotic and infective complications. It allows easy needling after a period of maturation and is readily assessable for patency on clinical grounds.

Large bore, double-lumen venous catheters (e.g. Vascath) still have a role to play in acute RRT, however, given their relatively high complication rates, they should only be used as a bridge whilst autogenous access is being established or if kidney function is likely to recover. The National Kidney Foundation Kidney Disease Outcomes Quality Initiative (NKF K/DOQI) has advocated an increase in the proportion of patients who use autogenous AVFs [1].

Despite their usual plethora of medical comorbidities most ESRD patients who require chronic vascular access can have this achieved without a general anaesthetic as a day case under local or regional anaesthesia.

Pre-operative Considerations

In all patients at risk of requiring haemodialysis in the future utmost care should be taken to preserve the forearm veins. Arguably these veins should be preserved in *all* patients in case of future requirement for chronic vascular access.

Patients and medical staff should be instructed to avoid venous cannulation or venesection in the arm where possible. If venous cannulation is necessary then this should be restricted to the veins on the dorsum of the hand or palmar aspect of the wrist [2]. Preferably this should be instituted as a general guideline across the hospital. Obviously if emergent access is required then this should be sited where possible, although it still may be possible to avoid the non-dominant forearm or antecubital fossa.

Peripherally inserted central cannulae (PICC) lines should be avoided in renal failure patients as they have a propensity to destroy the peripheral veins making AVF formation difficult if not impossible in that arm.

A functioning AVF is a lifeline and therefore should never be used for anything other than renal replacement therapy.

Vascular Access Planning

The K/DOQI guidelines which suggest the creation of an AVF 12 months prior to the anticipated commencement of dialysis. Our policy is more in keeping with the United Kingdom Vascular Society Guidelines which advocate creation of an AVF 16-24 weeks prior to dialysis thus avoiding the small possibility of an established fistula failing even before it has been used [3].

If dialysis is required urgently then this should be achieved using a double lumen venous catheter and if it is predicted that the patients renal function is not going to recover then autogenous vascular access should be constructed as soon as possible to allow the fistula to mature before the patient has to endure too many complications from their venous catheter.

Clinical History

Prior to embarking on AVF creation it is important to take a full clinical history. Renal failure patients often have a legion of medical comorbidities. Many are on antiplatelet medication or oral anticoagulation therapy. We do not routinely stop antiplatelets or oral anticoagulants and will proceed with surgery as long as the international normalised ratio (INR) is less than 2.5.

A history suggestive of arterial disease is also important. Claudication (upper limb as well as lower limb), cerebrovascular disease (stroke or transient ischaemic attack) or ischaemic heart disease should be specifically enquired about.

Special attention must be paid to any history of previous vascular access procedures, central venous lines or pacemakers. If possible the patients' case notes should be scrutinized for details about the above.

Clinical Examination and Special Investigations

In the era of ready access to advanced vascular imaging it is easy to overlook the importance of clinical assessment, however, careful clinical examination can yield a wealth of helpful information. Simple palpation of the radial artery at the wrist may reveal a non-pulsatile, hard, artery suggestive of severe vascular calcification rendering it inoperable. This is not uncommonly seen in ESRD. Allen's test should be performed prior to the construction of a forearm fistula to ascertain the completeness of the collateral circulation. Although not an absolute contra-indication to fistula formation, a positive Allen's test may alert the clinician to the risk of steal phenomenon and prompt further investigation or the choice of another site for access. It may be that the arterial supply could be improved by percutaneous intervention prior to fistula formation. The engorgement of head and neck veins may indicate a central venous problem which is not uncommon in renal patients who have had numerous central venous catheters. Again this may be amenable to percutaneous intervention prior to surgery. Examination of the arms may reveal thrombosed or phlebitic veins unsuitable for the construction of a fistula. The presence of varicosities may preclude the use of lower limb veins. It is also important to ascertain the general condition of the patient – are they fluid deplete or overloaded? Would the patient be able to tolerate lying flat for the procedure? It is technically challenging to perform this type of surgery in an underfilled patient with collapsed veins.

Contraindications to AVF Formation

There are few absolute contraindications to the formation of an AVF. Of course a definite and absolute contraindication is the lack of any suitable arteries or veins!

Active skin infection, venous stenoses or occlusions and peripheral arterial disease are all relative contraindications and can usually be identified and addressed pre-operatively. Commonly in renal failure patients (and especially in diabetic patients) the arteries are heavily calcified. Often surgery is possible in these situations with some modification of technique (e.g. the use of occlusion balloon catheters or tourniquet) however on occasion it may be preferable to abandon the procedure before opening the artery and moving to a more proximal (and hopefully less diseased) location.

In our experience, it is possible to construct a functioning fistula in most situations. It is important to remember, that although vascular access is sometimes required urgently, there are very few situations when it is not possible to spend some time optimizing a medically frail patient, treating active infections or performing percutaneous intervention for vascular stenoses or occlusions. If a patient is deemed to be too unfit even for a procedure under local anaesthesia then reconsideration should be given to the decision to consider long term renal replacement therapy.

Primary Access and the Preservation of "Venous Real Estate"

Arterio-venous fistulae often give many years of good service but they do not come with a lifetime guarantee. Inevitably a fistula will fail. It is important therefore (especially in the younger patient) to maximise the number of fistulae that can potentially be created. It is important to start as distally as possible and progress proximally with each access procedure thus preserving venous "real estate" for future use. Our preferred order of AVF creation is outlined in table 2.

Table 2. Preferential order of AVF construction in the upper limb

1) Snuff box fistula
2) Radio-cephalic fistula at the wrist (Consider also: ulno-basilic AVF)
3) Radio-cephalic in the forearm (maybe possible to construct several of these fistula sequentially in the forearm)
4) Brachio-cephalic in the ante-cubital fossa (Consider also deep perforating vein – Gracz fistula)
5) Transposed brachial vein AVF
6) Prosthetic brachio-basilic or brachio-axillary prosthetic loop fistula

This order is not prescriptive and must be tailored to each patient. Not every patient will have suitable anatomy for these procedures. The skill in vascular access surgery is improvisation.

The non-dominant upper limb is used first. This is to allow the possibility of self needling (home dialysis) in the fitter patient. It also affords the patient some ability to read, use a computer or perform other tasks whilst dialysing.

Secondary Access

In patients with prior failed fistulae, or in those with unsuitable arteries or veins in the forearm, there are numerous other sites in the body where vascular access can be secured. In our experience these fistulae rarely function as effectively as a well constructed primary upper limb fistula, however in some patients the available options are somewhat limited. The transposition of the long saphenous vein into the upper limb is well described in the literature but we have found the maturation of these fistula to be disappointing. Renal failure patients are predisposed to peripheral and coronary arterial disease and it may be that the long saphenous vein should be preserved to be utilised as a conduit for future possible bypass surgery.

It is important to always re-evaluate a patient fully before each new access procedure. Although a distal AVF may have failed, the high blood flow prior to failure may have opened up other veins that had previously been deemed too small to use or overlooked completely in a previous assessment.

The various options for secondary access are described in detail elsewhere in this book.

Prosthetic AVFs

The use of prosthetic grafts, where necessary, can also increase the available options and allow vascular access in some of these more complicated patients. In patients with no suitable vasculature for an autogenous AVF a prosthetic graft may allow a good fistula to be formed. Prosthetic graft fistulae have poorer primary and secondary patency rates and higher levels of infective complications, but they do have the advantage of requiring no period of maturation and, if required, can be needled almost immediately after construction [4]. This also means that fistulae do not need to be constructed months in advance and may be something to consider in patients with limited life expectancy.

Other indications for prosthetic AVF construction are in patients who have had previous AVFs that have failed for no obvious anatomical or surgical reason. The high flow through a prosthetic fistula may alleviate this problem.

When using prosthetic material we strongly advocate pre-procedural testing for methicillin resistant staphylococcus aureus (MRSA) by swabbing the nares, throat, axillae and groins. If the patient is found to be colonized then suitable MRSA eradication treatment should be prescribed. Antibiotics covering MRSA (Intravenous Vancomycin or Teicoplanin) are used routinely when prosthetic material is implanted.

Technique

The vast majority of primary autogenous AVFs can be constructed under local anaesthetic as a day case procedure. Patients therefore do not need to be kept nil by mouth. In the author's unit the procedure is performed on a dedicated day theatre list with staff accustomed to an awake patient. Our preference is not to perform the procedure immediately after dialysis because of the relative fluid depletion and venoconstriction that occurs following dialysis.

Prophylactic antibiotics are only administered when introducing prosthetic material or if there is an increased risk of wound infection (e.g. known MRSA positivity). Pulse oximetry is measured throughout the procedure. An anaesthetist is not routinely required. If a proximal or prosthetic fistula is required (requiring axillary block or general anaesthetic), or if the patient is of a higher operative risk then that patient would be treated on a routine operating list with an anaesthetist present with full monitoring equipment.

Surgical loupes are always worn when constructing fistulae in order to correctly place sutures in the often small anastomoses.

Anatomical Snuffbox (Figure 1)

Our preference is to construct the most distal fistula possible and the snuff-box AV fistula (between the cephalic vein and the radial artery) is possible in about half of the patients presenting for primary AVF construction [5, 6]. The patency is similar to that of a primary forearm fistula and we feel that even if the fistula fails, it does not compromise the construction of a forearm fistula.

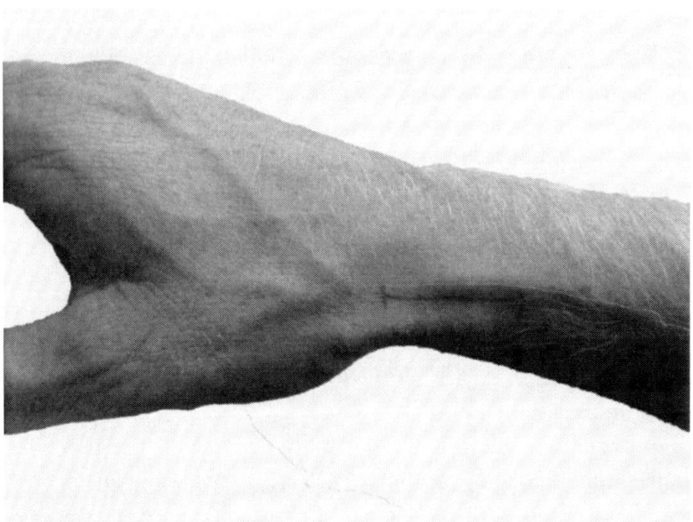

Blue: Cephalic vein and tributaries.
Red: Incision for snuffbox fistula.

Figure 1. Snuffbox fistula.

In fact a failed snuff-box fistula often simplifies the construction of a more proximal fistula and aids maturation of the more proximal fistula by arterializing the cephalic vein.

A longitudinal incision is made over the anatomical snuff box. The cephalic vein is identified subcutaneously and carefully dissected free. The dissection is carried deeper through the extensor retinaculum to expose the radial artery. There are often small branches from the deep surface of the radial artery which can be diathermized or divided between fine vicryl ligatures to allow the artery to be brought up into the wound. Our preference is to use elasticated slings passed twice around the artery proximally and distally to bring the vessel towards the surface and also to arrest flow through the isolated portion of the artery without using clamps. If control of bleeding cannot be achieved using the slings alone then small, soft vascular clamps (e.g. bulldog or Yasergil) may be applied.

The cephalic vein is ligated proximally and divided allowing sufficient length of vein to perform a tension-free end-to-side anastomosis onto the radial artery. The vein is flushed with heparinized saline and occluded distally to distend the vein. It is imperative that the vein is not twisted or kinked in its course. Occasionally some subcutaneous dissection can improve the course of the vein and superficializing it to some extent. The end of the vein is spatulated if necessary. A 3-4mm arteriotomy is made in the artery and the vein is anastomosed to the artery using a 6-0 polypropolene suture on an 11mm needle. Care is taken to create anastomosis big enough for a well functioning fisula but not so big as to risk a "steal" phenomenon with reverse flow in the distal artery. An anastomosis of no greater than 5mm will normally suffice.

Prior to closure of the anastomosis the vein and artery are unclamped, back-bled and flushed with heparinised saline. The inability to pass a small catheter through the anastomosis or difficulty in flushing the fistula should alert the clinician to a problem with the anastomosis or run off. The anastomosis is closed and the clamps removed. It can often be difficult to ascertain immediately if the fistula is functioning correctly. After a few minutes any spasm in the artery or vein should have subsided and a healthy fistula should have an easily palpable thrill in the vein with an associated machinery-like murmur. A sterilised stethoscope or hand held doppler is useful in assessing the fistula prior to closure of the skin. Pulsatility without a thrill or murmur often signifies a technical problem with the anastomosis or obstruction to the outflow. This could be thrombus (which may be treated by the passage of an embolectomy catheter) or an undiagnosed stenosis or obstruction downstream. It may be necessary to perform an on-table fistulogram in this situation.

Low Forearm (Brescia/Cimino)

A transverse incision is made antero-laterally in the forearm over a suitable segment of cephalic vein and radial artery (Figure 2).

The vein is dissected free and prepared in a similar fashion to the snuffbox fistula.

The radial artery is dissected free and controlled. An anastomosis is fashioned as per the snuffbox fistula. Occasionally it is necessary to partially divide brachioradialis muscle to allow passage of the cephalic vein medially without any significant tension or kinking.

The wounds are closed with a 3-0 absorbable subcuticular suture.

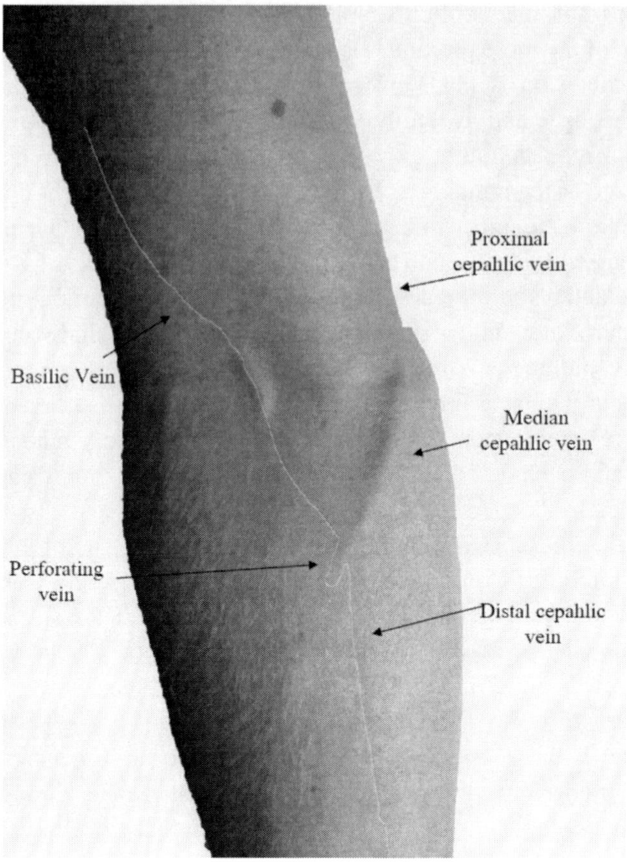

Figure 2. Forearm veins.

High Forearm

This is similar to the low forearm fistula, however it may be necessary to divide more muscle in order to get the vein to lie satisfactorily.

Upper Arm Radio- or Brachio-Cephalic Bypass

A transverse or "lazy S" incision is made across the upper part of the antecubital fossa. The cephalic vein is mobilized and prepared. It is necessary to mobilize a significant amount of vein as it has to be swung across the antecubital fossa to anastomose it without tension to the brachial artery.

The brachial artery is dissected free. It is often necessary to partially divide the bicipital aponeurosis, and if this is required it is vital to do this under direct vision in order not to damage the median nerve. The vein is anastomosed end-to-side with the artery as described above. When the fistula is functioning the wounds are closed with a subcuticular suture. We do not routinely use a drain.

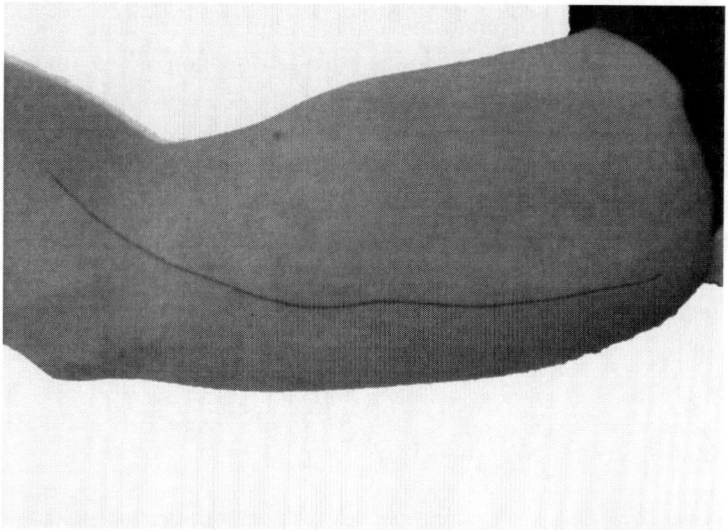

Blue continuous line: Basilic vein.
Blue dotted line: Position of basilic vein following transposition.
Red lines: Skin incisions.

Figure 3. Basilic vein transposition

A variation of this fistula is to utilise the deep perforating vein (Gracz fistula). This vein is often quite short and may require careful mobilization in order to secure enough length to construct a tension free anastomosis with the brachial artery (Figure 2).

Basilic Vein Transposition (Figure 3)

When previous distal AVFs have failed, or the native forearm vessels are and the cephalic vein is unsuitable (<3mm or obstructed) then it is necessary to utilize the basilic vein. When radio-cephalic and brachio-cephalic fistulae have failed or are not possible, brachio-basilic fistulae provide patency rates superior to prosthetic grafts [7].

In its anatomical position the basilic vein provides only a short segement that can be cannulated. The vein is often relatively deep and inaccessible. Therefore the course of the vein has to be altered in order to create a useful AVF.

The vein can be transposed as a 1- or 2-stage procedure. In our institution we prefer the single stage method, however both are described here. Although it is possible to perform this procedure under local anaesthesia, it is technically more challenging than a forearm fistula. Therefore in an anxious or less robust patient it may be desirable to perform this procedure under general anaesthesia.

One-Stage Basilic Vein Transposition

A longitudinal incision is made over the basilic vein in the upper arm. Given that a significant length of basilic vein needs to be mobilized (to just below the elbow) it is useful to make this incision as a series of interrupted cuts in order to facilitate wound healing. The basilic vein is then dissected free paying particular attention not to damage the medial cutaneous nerve of arm.

A separate transvers incision is made antero-medially, above the elbow crease and through this the brachial artery is dissected free and controlled. The brachial vein is transacted below the elbow and tunnelled antero-laterally over the belly of the biceps muscle. A paediatric feeding catheter can be passed up the vein when transposed to ensure no kinks or twists. It is also helpful to mark along the anterior surface of the vein with an indelible marker prior to tunnelling to aid orientation. The vein is prepared and anastomosed to the artery as described previously. The wounds are closed with subcuticular sutures.

Two-Stage Basilic Vein Transposition

A transvers incision is made antero-medially, just above the elbow crease. The basilic vein is anastomosed end-to side to the brachial artery using the aforementioned technique. The wounds are closed and then a period of 4-6 weeks is allowed for the vein to mature.

Following adequate maturation (assessed clinically and/or ultrasonographically), the patient reurns to theatre. A longitudinal incision is made over the basilic vein and this is dissected free and elevated to a more lateral subcutaneous plane. Alternatively the vein is transacted adjacent to the anastomosis, tunnelled antero-laterally and then re-anastomosed more proximally on the brachial artery. Again care is taken not to kink or twist the vein and the anastomosis is performed as described earlier. The wounds are closed with subcuticular sutures.

Post Operative Care

Following the procedure the arm is dressed with a simple, adherent dressing. It is often useful to wrap the limb in warm wool gauze (Gamgee), but circumferential or tight bandages must be avoided at all costs.

The fistula should be monitored every half an hour for the presence of a thrill or murmur and it is useful for the operating surgeon to mark on the dressing where the thrill is best felt and the murmur best heard prior to the transfer of the patient out of theatre. It may not be possible to initially feel a pulse distal to the fistula but the distal limb should be assessed for any change in movement or sensation, warmth and capillary refill which can indicate hypo-perfusion of the distal limb suggestive of steal phenomenon.

Again it is important that the blood pressure is monitored by a cuff on the contralateral arm and no attempts are made to cannulate the veins or venesect from the operated arm.

Patients are reviewed by renal access specialist nurses one week following surgery. Wounds are inspected and any sutures or skin clips are removed. Following this review, patients are encouraged to perform hand exercises such as squeezing of a squash ball to encourage fistula development and maturation. Depending upon the patient and renal physician the fistula should be ready for use in approximately six weeks from its formation.

REFERENCES

[1] III. NKF-K/DOQI Clinical Practice Guidelines for Vascular Access: update 2000. *Am. J. Kidney Dis.* 2001; 37(1 Suppl 1):S137-81.

[2] Gibbons CP. Primary vascular access. *Eur. J. Vasc. Endovasc. Surg.* 2006; 31(5):523-9.

[3] Winearls CG FR, Mitchel DC. The organization and delivery of the vascular access service for maintenance haemodialysis patients. *Report of a joint working party.* 2006.

[4] Perera GB, Mueller MP, Kubaska SM, et al. Superiority of autogenous arteriovenous hemodialysis access: maintenance of function with fewer secondary interventions. *Ann. Vasc. Surg.* 2004; 18(1):66-73.

[5] Wolowczyk L, Williams AJ, Donovan KL, Gibbons CP. The snuffbox arteriovenous fistula for vascular access. *Eur. J. Vasc. Endovasc. Surg.* 2000; 19(1):70-6.

[6] Bonalumi U, Civalleri D, Rovida S, et al. Nine years' experience with end-to-end arteriovenous fistula at the 'anatomical snuffbox' for maintenance haemodialysis. *Br. J. Surg.* 1982; 69(8):486-8.

[7] Gonzalez E, Kashuk JL, Moore EE, et al. Two-stage brachial-basilic transposition fistula provides superior patency rates for dialysis access in a safety-net population. *Surgery*; 148(4):687-93; discussion 693-4.

INDEX

A

B

C

D

E

F

G

H

I

J

K

L

M

N

O

P

T

U

V